How to read and critique research:

a guide for nursing and healthcare students

T0286601

Sara Miller McCune founded SAGE Publishing in 1965 to support the dissemination of usable knowledge and educate a global community. SAGE publishes more than 1000 journals and over 800 new books each year, spanning a wide range of subject areas. Our growing selection of library products includes archives, data, case studies and video. SAGE remains majority owned by our founder and after her lifetime will become owned by a charitable trust that secures the company's continued independence.

Los Angeles | London | New Delhi | Singapore | Washington DC | Melbourne

How to read and critique research:
a guide for nursing and healthcare students

Helen Aveyard
Nancy Preston
Morag Farquhar

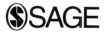

Los Angeles | London | New Delhi
Singapore | Washington DC | Melbourne

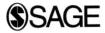

Los Angeles | London | New Delhi
Singapore | Washington DC | Melbourne

SAGE Publications Ltd
1 Oliver's Yard
55 City Road
London EC1Y 1SP

SAGE Publications Inc.
2455 Teller Road
Thousand Oaks, California 91320

SAGE Publications India Pvt Ltd
B 1/I 1 Mohan Cooperative Industrial Area
Mathura Road
New Delhi 110 044

SAGE Publications Asia-Pacific Pte Ltd
3 Church Street
#10-04 Samsung Hub
Singapore 049483

Editor: Laura Walmsley
Editorial assistant: Sahar Jamfar
Production editor: Sarah Cooke
Copyeditor: Sharon Cawood
Proofreader: Neil Dowden
Indexer: Silvia Benvenuto
Marketing manager: Ruslana Khatagova
Cover design: Sheila Tong
Typeset by: C&M Digitals (P) Ltd, Chennai, India
Printed in the UK

Library of Congress Control Number: 2022937422

British Library Cataloguing in Publication data

A catalogue record for this book is available from the British Library

ISBN 978-1-5297-3298-6
ISBN 978-1-5297-3297-9 (pbk)

At SAGE we take sustainability seriously. Most of our products are printed in the UK using responsibly sourced papers and boards. When we print overseas we ensure sustainable papers are used as measured by the PREPS grading system. We undertake an annual audit to monitor our sustainability.

Contents

About the authors

Dr Helen Aveyard is Principal Lecturer in the Oxford School of Nursing and Midwifery at Oxford Brookes University. After completing her undergraduate nursing degree, combining clinical duties with study, Helen completed her MA in Medical Law and Ethics and her PhD. On taking up an academic role, she has published widely on nursing ethics and education in research methods. Helen is an experienced supervisor for PhD and professional doctorate students, and is the author of *Doing a Literature Review in Health and Social Care* (2019), which is in its fourth edition. Other co-authored texts include *A Post-graduate's Guide to Doing a Literature Review* (2021) and *A Beginner's Guide to Evidence Based Practice* (2017), all published by Open University Press. Helen has written previous courses for Epigeum in 2010 and 2017.

Professor Morag Farquhar is Professor of Palliative Care Research at the University of East Anglia (UEA). An early graduate nurse by background (King's College London), she holds an MSc in Medical Sociology and a PhD (University of London). She has worked in health services research for over 30 years, predominantly in the field of supportive and palliative care, within the universities of London, Manchester, Cambridge and UEA. Her main research areas are person-centred care, informal carers, breathlessness in advanced disease, and the developing and testing of interventions using mixed methods. Morag has collaborated and published with colleagues internationally in the field of breathlessness in advanced disease and palliative care methodology. At UEA, Morag teaches on research and using evidence in clinical practice across a range of undergraduate and postgraduate health care professional programmes, including PhD supervision and examination.

Professor Nancy Preston is a Professor of Supportive and Palliative Care and an Associate Dean for Post Graduate Education in the Faculty of Health and Medicine at Lancaster University. She completed her degree in Nursing at King's College, London and worked as a cancer nurse, including time spent as a research nurse on clinical trials. She completed her PhD at the Institute of Cancer Research, London. With over 30 years of experience in research, Nancy's work focuses on palliative care and how best to integrate palliative care into general health care systems. She has a strong interest in how people make decisions about their future care, including advanced care planning and experiences around assisted dying. She has been involved in five European research projects and has published over 150 research papers. Nancy is an experienced PhD supervisor and examiner, and is the co-author of *A Post-graduate's Guide to Doing a Literature Review* (2021) and *Palliative Care Nursing* (2018).

Acknowledgements

We would like to thank the authors of the papers we included who generously gave their time to respond to the chapters. We would also like to thank Dr Frank Preston for creating the 'clips' from the papers.

Introduction

If you are reading this book, you have probably just embarked upon a nursing or health care course, have come across the frequent mention of terms such as 'research' and 'evidence-based practice', and are keen to find out what all this means in relation to your studies and clinical placements. You might be wondering why research is so important in nursing and health care when they are predominantly practical disciplines. Research underpins evidence-based practice, and this is a concept that you will be working with from the very beginning of your course, until qualification and beyond.

This book will help you to understand the research that informs the evidence base and the papers or articles (henceforth referred to as papers for consistency) that are published in academic journals reporting that research. It's a good idea if you can develop an understanding of this from the outset of your course, as your lecturers and practice educators will make frequent reference to research and evidence-based practice throughout your study. You are also likely to be asked to review (critically appraise) research papers as part of an assignment.

The problem is that research can seem daunting. Indeed, some of it is complex and there are many research papers that we would not recommend you start off with – there are also many papers that senior researchers disagree over and, again, we would not recommend engaging with these in the first instance. Even some of the simpler research papers might seem out of reach at first glance. Understanding the terms and concepts that you need to be familiar with before you get to grips with a paper will help you feel more confident when reading and reviewing it.

This is where the challenges lie. Given the importance of research-informed practice, it is essential that you are able to read, understand and discuss research papers from the beginning of your studies. This requires some knowledge of research and a critical eye. As a student, you need to develop these skills of reading, understanding and critiquing research as early as possible, so that you can confidently discuss the evidence (usually research papers) in your written work and in any presentations you give. There is no way forward other than starting to read research papers – some of which will be straightforward to understand, others less so.

We have written this book to help you to do this. As a student nurse or health care professional, you will come across a variety of research papers throughout your course and your clinical practice. In this textbook, we have identified some of the most common research designs and, for each, identified an example of a research paper that follows that design. We will walk you through each paper, pointing out key features and decisions that the researchers have made when conducting and reporting their research, so that you can follow the steps they have taken and understand their reasons.

We will also suggest different ways things could have been done. The aim is to help you read and understand papers with a confident critical eye. All of the papers identified are relevant to nursing practice; however, we are using the papers to illustrate a research method rather than to draw attention to the results of a specific paper – so we hope that these remain of interest to other health care students and professionals. We do hope, however, that, given the relevance of the research papers to health care, you will find the examples interesting and relevant, in addition to their main purpose here of acting as an example of a paper using a particular research method.

How this book is presented

Each chapter in this book presents a different research paper related to a different research method. In doing so, we will explore the most common research methods that you are likely to come across. Rather than discussing research concepts in an abstract way, we present presenting specific examples, in the form of research papers that are relevant to nursing and health care, that will help your understanding. The papers we have selected will be typical examples of papers that you might be asked to review within your course or come across in your clinical practice. We will then explore each paper in depth, using it as a springboard for discussion of the various research concepts and methods. This means that all of the discussion is directly relevant to what you might read in a paper; all the concepts are explored in relation to an actual research paper rather than discussed in isolation. We have annotated key aspects of the papers and presented them in the chapters to help you navigate the paper and enhance your understanding.

Text in these boxes are extracts from the research papers.

Where possible, we have followed the same format and used the headings for each chapter in terms of the key features and content we explore within each paper – this should help build your confidence as you work through the book, as you will see how many research concepts relate to, or are fundamental to, many seemingly varied research methods. If, rather than working through the book, you are exploring individual chapters to better understand a research design relating to a paper you are reading for your studies, the chapter structure and headings will help you work through this. The chapters and research designs (and therefore types of papers) included in this book are outlined below:

- Chapter 1: Getting started with reading research
- Chapter 2: A survey paper
- Chapter 3: A generic qualitative research paper

- Chapter 4: A grounded theory paper
- Chapter 5: A phenomenology paper
- Chapter 6: A randomised controlled trial paper
- Chapter 7: A case-control study paper
- Chapter 8: A mixed methods study paper
- Chapter 9: An integrative review paper
- Chapter 10: A systematic review with meta-analysis paper

How were the papers chosen?

The papers identified for this book were chosen as they all represent an example of the particular research method. The papers are not intended to be perfect examples of the methods identified: no paper ever is. We wanted to provide working examples of the research methods to help you identify key features to consider when reading other papers using that method. We therefore chose papers that we considered would provide a good learning opportunity. All of the papers we have used are open access which means they can be obtained online but without passwords, library login accounts or by paying an access fee – they are in the public domain for everyone. We strongly recommend that you access a copy of each paper to work through alongside reading each chapter.

We also contacted the authors of the research papers and asked them to comment on our chapter about their paper: our appraisal of it. In many instances, the researchers have contributed to the chapters and gave us their rationale for the steps they took; sometimes there was a rationale that could not be included in the paper due to the restricted word counts that journals need to apply. We are very grateful to these researchers for taking the time to do this and feel that this adds to the authenticity of the book.

We have tried to include contemporary papers in this book, although the date of a study is not an essential prerequisite for learning about research concepts and methods. It is also important to note that the time from conducting a study, to writing it up as a paper and submitting it to a journal, and then to actual publication can be quite lengthy. You can get a sense of this as researchers often report when data was collected, and some journals also report the submission date and acceptance date of manuscripts (i.e. when the paper has gone through peer review by other experts in the field, been revised in response to those reviews, and then finally been accepted by the journal editors for publication).

This book is an ideal resource for undergraduate students who are engaging with research for the first time. It is also intended as an introductory text for those studying at postgraduate level or those who are new to reading research papers. Further, it is an ideal text for practitioners who are returning to study or who are updating their skills in continuing professional development. This book will give you a step-by-step guide to understanding research, using real-world, relevant examples in an accessible way.

1 Getting started with reading research

Why is research important in nursing and health care?

Nursing and health care are both an art and a science. It is likely that this is a phrase that you have heard before because it is very hard to argue that they are one or the other. There is a science or evidence base that underpins clinical practice but there is also a human side which requires the art of caring, compassion and empathy. In practice, the two are intertwined; there is a science to caring as well as an art. However, it is the science aspect of nursing and health care that we are going to consider in this book: the research, and the evidence it produces, that underpins our practice.

When you attend a health care appointment, you will want to feel confident that the practitioner is using the best available evidence with which to make decisions about your care and treatment. For example, if you are planning an overseas trip to an area where malaria is prevalent, you would expect to receive appropriate advice about taking medication for the prevention of malaria. You may have heard about some unpleasant and even dangerous side-effects from some anti-malarial medication such as depression, panic attacks and even psychotic symptoms. These have been widely reported in the non-academic general press (for example, *The Guardian*, 2 June 2017). Given the nature of these symptoms, you would probably expect that the reported side-effects have been systematically reported and investigated. To make sense of any individual reports of serious side-effects, we need to see how many people are affected by them within a much larger sample of people taking the drug. We also need to monitor and follow up those affected in detail and see what other risk factors, if any, were present. This type of research is often undertaken using a case-control study, where those who have been exposed to a particular event or drug (in this case, anti-malarial tablets) are compared to those who have had no such exposure: the symptoms experienced by the people in both groups are then compared. This enables researchers to identify whether there is a higher number of symptoms in those who have been exposed to the event or drug. We discuss this type of study in Chapter 7. Crucially, you would also expect the clinician to be able to answer your questions in a knowledgeable and informed way; to do this, they need to be aware of, and have understood and considered the value of, the research which has investigated this.

In health care, it is very important that we don't draw conclusions from anecdotal evidence. A practice nurse might have a friend who suffered with side-effects from anti-malarial drugs and so tells his or her patients this, suggesting that they are not to be used. Yet, the evidence shows that they are safe when appropriately prescribed – certainly safer than contracting malaria. Therefore, the clinician who uses anecdotal or personal experience to inform their professional practice is not using evidence or delivering evidence-based practice.

BOX 1.1: A NOTE ON ANECDOTES

Consider how easy it is, in everyday life, to be tempted to draw conclusions from anecdotal evidence. It could be tempting to conclude from the general press, or from anecdotes from individuals, that all anti-malarial drugs are dangerous. Remember that anecdotes are just that – a one-off. In order to see if they are representative of a wider problem, we need to conduct systematic studies.

Health care should be based on the systematic observations drawn from the study of practice. It is hard to argue against this. The idea that practice should be based on research has a long history within health care. When it first appears as if there might be an association between two variables (factors such as diseases and risk factors), it is important that these are systematically investigated to see if there is a true relationship rather than an association being assumed. This is how scientists identified that smoking caused lung cancer. In this case, scientists identified a particular set of conditions that might have been associated with lung cancer. They were able to compare these conditions in people who had the disease and those who did not, and were able to identify that significantly more people who smoked went on to develop lung cancer; they were able to identify a likely correlation between the two (a relationship). As we will see later in this book, correlation does not necessarily mean causation, and so we always need to be careful about the conclusions we draw from studies where a correlation is found. If you would like to find out more about these studies, Cicco et al. (2016) have written a summary of the smoking and lung cancer studies that were undertaken.

Even back in the 1700s, Royal Navy doctor James Lind had a hunch of a correlation: he thought that if the diet of sailors was improved by including citrus fruit, the incidence of scurvy would be reduced. Rather than simply introducing such fruit into the diets of all those at sea, he decided to study this in a more systematic and controlled manner. Lind conducted what is often considered one of the first controlled experiments in health care. In this experiment, he introduced citrus fruit to one group of sailors, and withheld citrus fruit from another group. He then monitored their health to see if those who had been given the fruit had a lower incidence of scurvy. Careful observation of both groups identified that citrus fruit did indeed reduce the risk of scurvy. You might argue that if he had such a hunch that increasing citrus fruit in the diet would have such an effect, it was unethical to withhold the fruit from one group of people. This is a valid concern; however, we need to remember that Lind's initial hunch might not have been proved to be correct. Unless we study the effect of a possible intervention or care procedure carefully, we will never know for sure if (or why) it works.

Whilst we have a history of researching our practice since the time of the 1700s, it is also fair to say that our commitment to research and evidence-based practice has not always been consistent. Many people have commented that tradition, ritual and thinking along the lines of 'we have always done it this way' have dominated nursing and health care practice for a considerable time. Nowadays, there is a strong commitment to research within nursing and health care which has increased over the past few decades (Richards et al., 2018a, 2018b; Stolley et al., 2000; Tingen et al., 2009).

What is evidence-based practice?

The concept that practice should be based on research evidence has gradually evolved, and practitioners are increasingly concerned that the care they deliver is based on the strongest available evidence. This concept, known as evidence-based practice, has become the cornerstone of health care. Evidence-based practice has been defined as: 'The conscientious and judicious use of current best evidence in conjunction with clinical expertise and patient values to guide health (and social) care decisions' (Sackett et al., 2000: 71–2). From this definition, you can see that evidence-based practice is not just about evidence alone. Using an evidence-based approach to our care includes considering the preference of the patient and using our professional judgement. Patient preference and informed consent prior to care and treatment is a concept that you will consider in your teaching on law and ethics (Ellis, 2020). Professional judgement is something that you will develop as you gain experience. We will not be focusing further on either of these two concepts within this book; however, it is important that you are aware of them. In this book, we will focus on the 'research evidence' component of evidence-based practice. This is the central concept of this book and it is within this context that we will be exploring research. It is also important to note that research is not always available on a topic (Aveyard and Sharp, 2017): in this case, professional judgement becomes more important.

Does research always follow a gap in evidence?

Prior to a research study, researchers need to establish what is currently known about the topic they are interested in. There is little point in repeating a study if it has already been done (and this can also be unethical), although this depends on the size and quality of the earlier study and whether the results can be considered to be generalisable: that is, applicable to populations outside the study itself. For this reason, a short literature review will usually be included in the introduction to a study, which forms a summary of the existing knowledge in the area and hence justification for the study that is being reported. In addition, researchers will also often contact members of the public who have an interest in the research area to discuss the research with them. In the UK, this is usually referred to as patient and public involvement (PPI), public involvement in research or service user input. These consultations can be undertaken at various stages of the project, from establishing the rationale for the project, to its design, analysis and implementation and interpretation: they are an essential component of the research. When you are reading a study, do look out for evidence of involvement from members of the public or service users.

Research, audit or service evaluation

You might come across discussion about whether a project is research or audit or service evaluation. In broad terms, if the study aims to have generalisable or transferable findings, then it is classified as research, whereas if the results are for local use only, it might be classified as audit (for example, asking a question about whether the service meets a certain standard) or service evaluation (does the service meet an acceptable standard of care?). Research answers questions about what should be done, audit examines if it is being done (and if not, why not) and service evaluation explores the impact of care on experience outcomes. Twycross and Shorten (2014) have a useful paper describing the differences.

There are two main reasons why the distinction is important: one is that the robustness of project design can vary between the three, and the other is that the way a project is classified can affect the regulatory procedures that surround it, with research having more onerous regulatory requirements than audit or service evaluation. The boundaries between these types of studies can be a little blurred but there are some helpful tools to help you decide, such as one from the UK's Health Research Authority (found at www.hra-decisiontools.org.uk/research).

How do I recognise research?

Research is usually written up as a scientific paper and published in an academic journal. These journals can be accessed online or in a bound copy in an academic library. Publications in academic journals are often considered to be the gold standard for practitioners because the material has been peer reviewed and rigorously checked before publication. Some practitioner journals also publish research papers and use a peer-review process, but not all.

There are many types of research that inform our nursing and health care practice. In this book, we discuss different research approaches, designs and methods. We use the term empirical research in this book when we are referring to research studies that have collected data (either by observation or measurement of something), analysed that data and drawn conclusions from it; this is sometimes also called primary research. The papers presented in Chapters 2–8 of this book are empirical studies. By contrast, literature reviews collect together the findings of a group of relevant empirical studies, analyse them and draw conclusions from them. The papers presented in Chapters 9 and 10 of this book are literature reviews. Empirical research therefore collects data directly, rather than using data collected from previous research as a review does.

Whilst all types of research have distinct features, there are also core similarities which enable you to identify a piece of scholarly work as 'research'. First of all, you would expect to see a **research question or an aim**. These terms are often used interchangeably: they essentially mean the same thing but are structured differently (a research question is formed as a question, whereas an aim is formed as a sentence or statement). The research question or aim is often supplemented by objectives which are narrower, focused goals that the researchers are trying to achieve within their overall study: the steps required to answer the question or address the aim. The research question or aim usually follows from a consideration of the existing research that has been undertaken in an area; that is, existing work should be described in detail in a section outlining the background literature – it should identify the knowledge gap that the study aims to fill.

Once you have noted the research question or aim and the knowledge gap in the background literature, all research should have a clearly documented **methods section**. This is the section of the paper where the researchers report what they did in order to answer their research question, or address their aim, and why. The methods section might refer to the term **methodology** which is the rationale for the methods. The terms methods and methodology are sometimes used interchangeably but they do have different meanings. You might also come across mention of the **paradigm** within which the research is located. Put simply, a paradigm is the worldview within which research is located. For many years, the dominant paradigm within science was the positivist paradigm. This is associated with testing ideas through deductive quantitative methods. The classic experiment is an example of research that is located in a positivist paradigm. Researchers develop an intervention and give it to one group of people whilst withholding it from another. The outcomes of the two groups are then measured and compared at the end of the experiment – just as James Lind did. Over time, it became apparent that not all research questions, especially those within nursing and health care, could be answered through such deductive methods and more exploratory methods were developed. For example, trying to understand patients' experiences of an illness or intervention cannot easily be explored through a positivist, deductive method. These alternative methods sit within a constructivist paradigm.

There are many more paradigms and we could discuss these further, but, for simplicity, we are taking the approach in this book that most nursing and health care research can be categorised into either the positivist or the constructivist paradigm. Furthermore, within these paradigms, most research can be categorised as being either quantitative or qualitative in its approach. These are umbrella terms embracing a range of methods and are commonly used within nursing and health care. In broad terms, the positivist paradigm usually uses quantitative research designs: designs that enable the counting and measuring of results; for example, how many student nurses access a particular nursing journal online every month. These results can be clearly recorded and reported as a numerical measurement. There are different types of quantitative designs and we have included three examples within this book (in Chapters 2, 6 and 7). The constructivist paradigm usually uses qualitative research designs: designs that enable a rich description that illuminates, rather than quantifies, the phenomenon under study – for instance, why students accessed, or didn't access, a particular journal. These answers are likely to be in-depth and rich in content: more suited to exploration and discussion than to numerical measurement. There are different types of qualitative designs and we have included three examples within this book (in Chapters 3, 4 and 5). Some studies incorporate both qualitative and quantitative methods within them and are referred to as mixed methods studies (we explore a mixed methods paper in Chapter 8). Other studies that identify, review and synthesise existing research on a topic are referred to as literature reviews. There are different types of literature review and we have included two examples within this book (in Chapters 9 and 10).

In addition to these overarching paradigms of positivism and constructivism and types of research, such as qualitative, quantitative, mixed methods or literature review, you are likely to find that the method is further defined with the **name of a particular method**. Qualitative and quantitative approaches are umbrella terms covering different methods. As we've seen, the approach taken depends on the research question or aim of the study – the same is true for the method, or methods, used within that approach. The research question or aim should drive the selection of the approach and guide the selection of a method. For example, if you are interested in understanding the experiences of a particular group of patients (perhaps in order to develop an intervention to better support them), you would probably identify a qualitative approach and method as being more appropriate than a quantitative one; whereas, if you wanted to know how often, and to what level of severity, patients experienced a particular symptom, you would probably use a quantitative approach and method. Although methods are normally attributable to either the positivist or constructivist paradigm, and the method is likely to be either qualitative or quantitative, these distinctions can sometimes become blurred. For example, an experiment is always positivist/quantitative and a grounded theory study always constructivist/qualitative, but whilst a survey is usually quantitative, there are some examples of surveys which collect qualitative data (or both quantitative and qualitative data). In this book, we therefore discuss a range of methods including: **surveys, randomised controlled trials and case-control studies**, as examples of **quantitative methods, and generic qualitative research, grounded theory, phenomenology** as examples of **qualitative methods**. A **mixed methods study** is reviewed and **literature reviews** as a research method are also presented.

You might hear discussion about a 'hierarchy of evidence' in which research methods are ranked in a hierarchy or an order. This term implies that the higher up the hierarchy a methodology is located, the stronger the evidence it produces is assumed to be. One of the first hierarchies of evidence, developed by Sackett et al. (1996), ranks the strength of evidence regarding how effective a treatment or an intervention is. This hierarchy of evidence *for determining effectiveness* is set out in the following order, starting with the strongest evidence:

- systematic reviews of randomised controlled trials (RCTs)
- RCTs
- cohort studies, case-control studies
- surveys
- case reports
- qualitative studies
- expert opinion
- anecdotal opinion.

In this hierarchy, studies are ranked according to their risk of bias. Studies that are very controlled (such as RCTs, which we discuss in Chapter 6) are usually considered to have a lower risk of bias and so are placed higher up in the hierarchy compared to those that are less controlled. The term hierarchy of evidence can be confusing. It might seem to imply that some forms of evidence are 'better' than others. However, this is not the case. Instead, studies with a low risk of bias are higher up the hierarchy. Yet, such very controlled studies with a low risk of bias, such as RCTs, can only be used to answer very specific research questions: they cannot be used to answer all research questions. The hierarchy of evidence is specific to research questions about effectiveness and does not equate with the concept of identifying the most appropriate method for the research question or aim. Therefore, the term hierarchy of evidence can be misleading as it is tempting to think that those methods at the top of the hierarchy will *always* be preferable to those further down it. Given that qualitative methods are generally at the bottom of the hierarchy of evidence (simply because they are not highly controlled), it could be tempting to question whether these are suitably rigorous methods for research. The answer is that qualitative methods are an appropriate – and indeed *the* most appropriate – method for answering questions that require the in-depth exploration and investigation of a phenomenon, regardless of where they sit within the hierarchy of evidence.

All methods should be clearly described and attributed to a named approach. Often, the type of study you are reading is given in the title of the paper; if not, it will certainly be explained in the methods section. The methods section of a study will report the full details of how the study was undertaken. For example, if the research reports an experiment, you should see the full details, described step by step, as an account of how the experiment was conducted and analysed. If the research reports a phenomenological study using interviews, you should see details of how the interviews were designed, conducted and analysed. Writing in the 'first person' is sometimes used here – for example, *'we did this...'* – which emphasises the tasks and activities undertaken by the researchers in the project, such as how the study was designed, conducted and analysed.

The methods section will be followed by **results** or **findings**. This is the section where papers reporting on studies involving different research approaches and methods can vary a lot. For quantitative research papers – those which collect and report numerical results – the results may include tables and graphs as well as the use of text to present the results. Descriptive statistics describe the study findings. In broad terms, the purpose of quantitative research is to undertake research on a representative sample and to generalise the results from this sample to the wider population. It is the use of inferential statistics that enable us to make this generalisation. Inferential statistics provide a numerical estimate about whether it is possible to apply the findings to the wider population. The results of both the descriptive data analysis and the accompanying statistical tests are usually accompanied by a written narrative explaining what the tables or graphs show.

Qualitative research papers – those which do not draw on numerical measurement but focus on the collection and reporting of a textually rich narrative – will report a synthesis of the grouped findings of the narrative data, such as interviews that have been conducted for the study. This is sometimes referred to as a thematic analysis. The grouped findings are often reported as themes or categories and often include examples of extracts from the data to illustrate them, such as quotes from interviews. It is therefore not unusual for qualitative research papers to be much longer than quantitative ones because of the additional text. Qualitative data is not interpreted using statistics – except for the inclusion of descriptive statistics about the general demographics of the sample – as the purpose of the analysis is not to generalise from a sample but to shed light on an area in an exploratory way. However, the reader may still consider the findings relevant and transferable to their area of practice. A mixed methods paper will present a combination of qualitative and quantitative results, and literature reviews will present the summary analysis of the literature included in the paper – depending on the type of review, this can be a narrative (qualitative) or may include quantitative analysis of the combined findings of the studies reviewed.

The results or findings section will be followed by a **discussion**. The discussion section is an exploration of what the results or findings might mean, particularly in the context of existing knowledge. Researchers will often draw on relevant theories, other research or policies to provide this context. The discussion section usually also considers the strengths and limitations of the study and suggests next steps or any unanswered questions that remain following the study, or new questions that arise from the study. Finally, papers usually include a **conclusion** – an overarching statement that synthesises the key findings and their implications (why they matter).

Was the study ethical?

All studies should mention how they safeguarded the rights of those involved through a consideration of **ethical principles**. You can find out about the ethical issues involved in Ellis (2020). It is always important to consider the ethics of any study. You might be tempted to think that if a study is published in a reputable, peer-reviewed journal then all the ethical considerations have been taken care of. This is very likely to be the case, as it is standard practice for studies within health care to be subject to scrutiny by an ethics committee prior to their commencement. However, this is not the case in all countries and, furthermore, ethical issues are rarely clear cut – you therefore might come across studies for which you feel unsure about the approach taken.

The ethics review is managed differently in different countries but generally consists of the identification and mitigation of possible ethical issues that might arise as a result of the study or study participation. In health care, it is usually done by a committee or a group of experienced researchers, clinicians and lay people (often including patients and informal carers). It is usually referred to as a research ethics committee and linked to the health service system. Depending on the type of study, the type of participants or how they were recruited, some studies report securing approval from university ethics committees.

The main reference point for those doing research is the Declaration of Helsinki (2013). This declaration, originally developed in 1964, was a direct response to the atrocities committed in the Second World War regarding involvement in research. These principles outline the standards of ethical research and provide guidance for the ethical conduct of research. We can also draw on the four principles of medical ethics, as developed by Beauchamp and Childress (2001), as a framework for the ethical consideration of research. These principles are autonomy (self-rule), beneficence (do good), non-maleficence (do no harm) and justice (do the right thing for all). For the review of research, we argue that the principles of autonomy (self-rule) and non-maleficence (do no harm) are often the most relevant. Beneficence (do good) can be challenging to apply to those research studies where the aim is to benefit future populations rather than those participating in the study: hence, its counterpart, non-maleficence, is the more practical principle. Justice is a broad principle and applies to the overall allocation of resources, including those given to research. This is an important principle but beyond the scope of this book, in which we are reviewing studies that have already been completed. Hence, when reviewing the research in each chapter, we will focus our ethical considerations on the principles of autonomy and non-maleficence.

The main application of the principle of autonomy is to ensure that potential participants are fully informed about the research project before they take part and are given a choice as to whether they wish to do so. It is important that potential participants do not feel any obligation to take part. For this reason, some form of information is given to the participant before they decide whether to take part. This provides an opportunity for the participant to consider whether or not they wish to take part in the research, or what questions they might like to ask before deciding. Participants should give their consent to take part only after they have been informed of what the study is about, as well as the potential risks and benefits of taking part: this is informed consent. They should also be given the opportunity to ask any questions they might have, and have them answered in a satisfactory way. Those who agree to take part are usually asked to sign a consent form.

Researchers also need to ensure that the informed consent of the participant to enter the study is genuine and free from coercion. It is important to consider that patients and staff might feel a duty to cooperate, and might fear that if they don't participate in a study it may affect their ongoing care (GMC, 2013) or ongoing relationships with colleagues. If a patient in hospital is approached by a member of the clinical team and asked if they would like to participate in a research study, it may be hard to say no, therefore every effort should be made to ensure that the patient does not feel obliged to enter a study. The same principle applies to members of staff who might feel obliged to participate in a study conducted in their place of work.

Associated with this is the consideration that the participant has the right to leave the study at any time. Currently, the Declaration of Helsinki (2013) states that participants in research have the right to leave without providing any reason for doing so. The justification for this is clear – if participants have a right to consent to involvement in a study, that right continues throughout the study and, by implication, includes the right to withdraw. However, the implications of withdrawal from a study also need to be considered. The involvement of participants in a study until its completion ensures there is sufficient data for the final analysis. For example, when researchers are following up on those who have entered a study, especially those that run over a period of time (such as some randomised controlled trials, as we discuss in Chapter 6), a high withdrawal rate will affect the quantity of data obtained and could even impact on confidence in the representativeness of the sample or strength of relationships in the findings. Hence, there is a balance to be struck between informing participants that withdrawing from a study is undesirable, whilst reaffirming their right to do so. Equally, in qualitative studies, once interviews are transcribed and the data has been used in the analysis, it can be difficult for researchers to disentangle the data of any individual who wishes to withdraw from a study. Participants are therefore often warned that, after a certain time point, it might be practically impossible to remove their data, although their active involvement in the study would have ceased.

Another ethical principle relating to research is the duty of non-maleficence: that is, do no harm. As in life, no research is risk free, but it is important to consider this as the purpose of research is usually to benefit future patients rather than the participating patients (even though participants may benefit). The participant needs to be aware that they are agreeing to take part in something that could cause harm. Harm can result from the inconvenience associated with involvement in the study or the study itself, or more direct harms – for instance, some studies involve the testing of new drugs where side-effects are unknown. Other studies involve participating in interviews which might reignite painful memories. However, we should not forget that there can be indirect benefits from taking part in a study. Participants might experience a sense of well-being from sharing their experiences and contributing to the greater good. In fact, some research does indicate that those participating in a research project do fare better than those who do not, probably due to the extra attention they receive from research staff (Nijjar et al., 2017).

How generalisable or transferable are the research findings?

The purpose of doing research in nursing and health care is to inform our practice and improve patient care and service delivery. It stands to reason that we cannot include everyone in a research study, instead we have to be selective. We carry out a study on a smaller group of people in the hope that the results can inform the care of many more. Therefore, who is included in the study is an important consideration: it impacts on the generalisability or transferability of the research. The term generalisability is associated with quantitative research, where the aim is to generalise the findings to the wider population. For qualitative research, the findings are not generalisable in a statistical way but they are likely to be transferable to other, similar patient groups or settings. One main factor contributing to the generalisability or transferability of the research findings is the representativeness of the sample.

All research is undertaken on a sample of people who are invited to participate, or a sample of records or events. The sample should be generally representative of the wider population but is, by definition, far smaller than the entire population. This is an important concept because if the sample does not reflect the wider population, then we should be cautious about drawing conclusions from it that we want to apply to the entire population. The extent to which it is possible to generalise from the sample in the study to a wider population is one of the main considerations of research. If we cannot draw conclusions from the study that can be generalised or that are transferable, then it begs the question why the research was undertaken in the first place. You might be tempted to think that the larger the sample the better. Yet, in reality, large samples might consist of people with certain characteristics who do not reflect the wider population, for example a limited age range, meaning that the results cannot be easily applied to other age groups. In general terms, quantitative research aims to have larger representative samples from which results can be generalised to the wider population, using statistical tests. Qualitative research tends to have smaller samples from which statistical generalisation is not possible, nor indeed desired, as the aim of qualitative research is to achieve depth of understanding; hence, the term transferability is often used to illustrate that concepts identified from qualitative research may be transferred to different contexts.

BOX 1.2: WHAT IS A SAMPLE?

An example of a sample is people who took part in a one-question survey that is sometimes conducted outside a polling station at an election (often referred to as an 'exit poll'). A sample of voters are asked how they voted as they leave the polling station and the findings are then used to predict the election result in news reports, often with surprising accuracy. You can imagine that the time of day the exit poll was conducted might impact on the type of answers gained as different types of people vote at different times of the day: office workers are unlikely to vote during office hours and they may vote differently to people who are unemployed or retired. However, the concept of an exit poll provides a useful illustration of sampling in research as such polls are not carried out at every voting station. Sampling involves identifying a selection of the population of interest who should represent the whole population of interest, thus enabling their views or results to be generalised or applied to that wider population. This is a concept we will return to throughout this book.

What is the difference between theory and research?

Earlier in this chapter, we outlined how to recognise a research paper: this is an important skill to achieve. It is also important to recognise other types of academic literature when you are reading within your discipline, in nursing or health care, and to understand how these relate to research. It is easy to feel overwhelmed when you are looking at nursing and health care literature as there are so many types of articles: research papers, discussion papers, opinion pieces, editorials, and so on. This is why it is important to recognise research but also the other types of literature you might come across. Discussion papers, for example, might refer to research but they are not research papers in their own right.

One concept that is important to understand is theory. The term 'theory' means different things to different people so you will find this term used in different ways. Sometimes we use it loosely and might say, '*I have a theory about why that man was murdered*'. In this case, theory is speculation. Other theories are far more developed and refer to a detailed explanation about the way things happen, or are expected to happen, often based on systematic observations. Take, for example, Darwin's theory of evolution, written after he studied the way in which animals and humans seem to have evolved. You will be aware that this theory is often challenged and, without concrete evidence to confirm it, it remains just a theory. We do not know for certain that humans evolved the way that is explained by Darwin's theory. Often in health and social care, a theory is developed as a result of research findings but is subject to amendment and refinement as different research findings become available. For example, Prochaska and colleagues (1994) developed a well-known theory often referred to as the 'stages of change model'. The authors developed a theory, based on research evidence, about the way in which people change their behaviour. This theory of behaviour change became very popular and much used by those whose role it was to help people stop smoking, lose weight or any other behaviour change that would promote a healthier lifestyle. However, as further evidence came to light, the stages identified in the theory were challenged (see, for example, West and Brown, 2013), and other researchers have not found strong evidence that the stages of behaviour change are as clear cut as originally postulated. This illustrates how theories are not static but change as new evidence arises. For a concise summary of theories, you might like to look at: www.sciencedirect.com/topics/psychology/middle-range-theory

Theories are different from research: they are overriding concepts about how things (might) work. Robust theories are underpinned by research. It is often proposed that qualitative research develops theory whilst quantitative research tests it. In practice this is a simplification, although it is true that qualitative research generates ideas whilst quantitative research is closely associated with the testing of them. Therefore, when you read a research paper, do consider the role of theory within it. As quantitative research usually tests theories, you might find these discussed in the introduction of the paper. In qualitative research, which is more exploratory, you might not come across any discussion of theory until the discussion section of the paper. Some qualitative research, such as grounded theory (which we discuss in Chapter 4), is explicitly designed to develop theory.

How do I find research and other evidence?

Research is generally published in academic journals which are most often accessed online – although many libraries do hold printed editions. If you know the reference for the research paper you are looking for, you can access this directly through the journal as the reference contains specific information about its location in the edition of the journal in which the paper is published (e.g. the volume, issue and page numbers).

When you do not have a specific paper or reference to look for, you can search for published research through an academic database which indexes papers published in many journals. Within nursing, one main database is CINAHL: the Cumulated Index to Nursing and Allied Health Literature. CINAHL is a database indexing a vast amount of research published in academic journals related to nursing and allied health care. There are other databases that can also be relevant; for example, Psycinfo is a database which indexes research published in academic journals which has a psychological health focus, so might be relevant to nursing, and MEDLINE is a database which has a more generic medical focus. You will find information when you access each database about the journals which are included. If you search different databases, you are likely to find that there is crossover in the journals that are covered by each – so the same paper can come up on a search of different databases. Google Scholar is another resource and, common to the main databases, shows whether a paper is accessible; for example, whether it is open access. Some journals, and some papers within journals, are open access (i.e. they do not need a password, library login or fee payment). You can sometimes get a more simply formatted version of a paper (e.g. as a pdf of a Word document) on an author's university website as some journals permit authors to upload these for public access after a certain period of time. Each database that you use is indexed using keywords by which you can identify the relevant research papers. Most databases use the concept of Boolean operators AND/OR to retrieve papers. The process of searching is described in Chapters 9 and 10. We recommend that you access training provided by your academic library in order to make the best use of the databases you need to use.

What is the range of nursing and health care research I might come across?

There is a wide range of nursing and health care research. In this book, we present just a selection of the most common of these. We discuss a survey, an experiment (we discuss randomised controlled trial) and a case-control study as examples of quantitative research. We discuss a generic qualitative research paper, a phenomenology and grounded theory paper as examples of qualitative research, and we discuss a mixed methods paper and two types of literature review.

SUGGESTED READING

Ellis, P. (2020) *Understanding Ethics for Student Nurses: Transforming Nursing Practice* (3rd edition). London: Sage Publications.

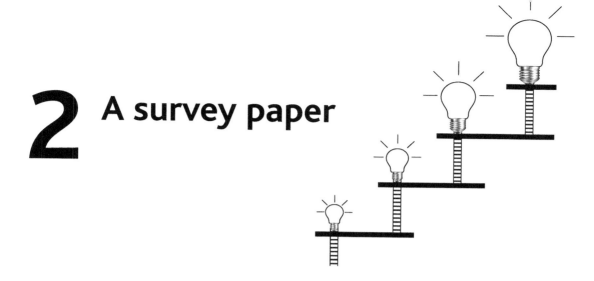

2 A survey paper

What is a survey?

We are all familiar with surveys. You will have been invited to complete them on many occasions. You might have been stopped on the street and asked for your views on a topic or given a questionnaire at the end of a lecture. You might have been enticed by an online retailer to 'take part in our survey', with the promise of a prize for a lucky winner. As surveys are part of our everyday lives, they are likely to be a method with which you are familiar, and which is intuitively easy to understand, and so we have devoted the first of our method-specific chapters of this book to them. However, they can be more complex than you might at first think, and in this chapter we will explain why this can be and what things you should look out for.

The term 'survey' is generic and can refer to the surveillance of any aspect of life – physical, behavioural, emotional, and so on. A survey can collect views and opinions or can simply involve counting or identifying what is there: people, animals, plants, infrastructure, and so on – for example, a survey of the drainage system in a local area. A general election is a type of survey. But, within health care, a survey typically takes the form of a questionnaire consisting of a pre-designed set of questions for which answers are sought from a representative group of people.

The survey paper we will explore in this chapter is:

Perry, L., Lamont, S., Brunero, S., Gallagher, R. and Duffield, C. (2015) The mental health of nurses in acute teaching hospital settings: A cross-sectional survey. *BMC Nursing*, 14(1): article no. 15.

Get yourself a copy of the paper. This is an open-access paper, as are all the papers we focus in on in the coming chapters. This means that you can access the paper freely online, without going through your university or hospital library account.

> Get yourself a copy of the paper, read it through, then work/read through the rest of the chapter, finding the points we identify in the paper: https://link.springer.com/article/10.1186/s12912-015-0068-8
>
> Scan the QR code to be taken straight to the paper.

What does the abstract and information about the authors tell me?

The first thing you come across when you read a paper, after the title, is the abstract. The abstract should be a standalone summary of the paper – it helps the reader judge whether the paper might be relevant to them or their needs. Most abstracts are structured with a set of sub-headings, but some are simply a paragraph – it all depends on the journal. Perry et al.'s (2015) abstract is structured.

In their abstract, Perry et al. (2015) give a concise summary of their study. It is clear from the abstract what the rationale was for the study. The methods are summarised and the headlines from the results are clearly presented. The researchers were interested in understanding the mental health of nurses in an acute hospital setting in Australia; they wanted to obtain a 'snapshot' insight into this important topic, and they used a survey to achieve this.

ABSTRACT

Background

Nursing is an emotionally demanding profession and deficiencies in nurses' mental well-being, characterised by low vitality and common mental disorders, have been linked to low productivity, absenteeism and presenteeism. Part of a larger study of nurses' health, the aim of this paper was to describe the mental health status and related characteristics of nurses working in two acute metropolitan teaching hospitals.

Methods

A cross-sectional survey design was used.

The Registered and Enrolled Nurse workforce, employed on any form of contract, at two teaching hospitals in Sydney, Australia were invited to participate.

The survey tool was compiled of validated tools and questions. Family and medical history and health risk-related characteristics, current psycho-active medications, smoking status, alcohol intake, eating disorders, self-perceived general health, mental health and vitality, demographic, social and occupational details were collected.

Results

A total of 1215 surveys were distributed with a usable response rate of 382 (31.4%). Altogether 53 nurses (14%) reported a history of mental health disorders, of which n = 49 (13%) listed diagnoses of anxiety and/or depression; 22 (6%) were currently taking psychoactive medication. Symptoms that could potentially indicate a mental health issue were more common, with 248 (65.1%) reporting they had experienced symptoms sometimes or often in the last 12 months.

Nurses had better mental health if they had better general health, lived with a spouse/partner rather than alone, had fewer symptoms, sleep problems or disordered eating behaviours, were not an informal carer and did not work nights. Nurses had greater vitality if they were male, had better general health, fewer sleep problems or symptoms generally and lived with a spouse/partner rather than alone; less vitality if they were an informal carer or had disordered eating.

Conclusion

Nurses and their managers should strive to create workplaces where working practices promote nurses' health and well-being, or at least are configured to minimise deleterious effects; where both nurses and their managers are aware of the potential for negative effects on the mental health of the workforce; where cultures are such that this can be discussed openly without fear of stigma or denigration.

Keywords: Absenteeism, Anxiety, Common mental disorder, Depression, Nurses, Nursing workforce, Mental health, Presenteeism, Vitality

Do look carefully at who the authors of the paper were. Understanding who undertook the research, and its cultural context, can tell you a lot about the paper. If the topic is something that you consider to be culturally specific, you might be less confident in applying findings of research that was undertaken in a different context. Alternatively, you might decide that cultural context is less important. You might also be interested in where the researchers work: the geographical location or type of institution.

The authors (Perry et al., 2015) were from Australia where the research was undertaken. It would be interesting to know from the paper whether the research team worked at, or had associations with, the hospitals involved in the study, and what the implications of this might be for how the study was run, and the effect this might have on the study findings and interpretation.

Is there a clear research question or aim addressed by the research?

The first question to ask of all research that you read is whether there is a research question or aim that is clearly and unambiguously stated near the beginning of the paper (before the methods are described). A research paper will have a title and sometimes an overriding statement, but this is different from a research question or aim: research questions or aims should be both very specific and explicit. You should look for an explicit question or aim that tells you the exact focus of the research.

Perry et al. (2015) have an explicit aim for their study:

METHODS

Aim

Part of a larger study of nurses' health, the aim of this component was to determine the mental health status and related characteristics of nurses working in two acute metropolitan tertiary referral hospitals in Sydney, Australia.

You will often find the aim or research question at the end of the background section in the main paper, or at the beginning of the methods sections – as Perry et al. (2015) have done. The aim or research question will not give you the method by which the researchers intend to answer the question, but it should provide a clear guide as to the focus of the study.

How was the study designed?

A survey is a snapshot of a situation at one point in time. Perry et al. (2015) wanted to determine the mental health status and related characteristics of nurses working in two acute hospitals in Australia, at a fixed time point. In this study, they were not investigating how the nurses' mental health or related characteristics changed over time: that would be a different, more complex study. So, Perry et al. (2015) conducted a cross-sectional survey, which collects data once, at one specific point in time: this reflects the stated aim of their study. We will discuss later on what the limitations of this approach are. If the authors had wanted to look at changes over time, they would have collected data at two or more time points – this would be called a longitudinal or follow-up study.

When you read a paper about a study that used survey methods, the first thing to consider is how the questionnaires and questions in it were designed. Questionnaires are not easy to design: their instructions and individual questions are not easy to write. Developed in haste, they can be confusing for the reader and result in the recording of information which is neither reliable nor useful. They can also result in low response rates due to the non-return of surveys and/or missing data, with some questions being left unanswered. This can lead to bias in the results, so questionnaires need to be developed carefully.

Questions might be developed using evidence from existing research or from exploratory interviews with a relevant population which is representative of the one being targeted. If it is a questionnaire for patients, then the developed questionnaire might then be commented on by members of the public who have experience or knowledge of the topic the questionnaire addresses (this is sometimes called Patient and Public Involvement, or PPI). It then needs to be tried out on a small group of people first (who are similar to those who will ultimately complete it), and then revised if need be, before it is ready to be used: this is often called piloting.

The concepts of validity and reliability are often discussed in relation to questionnaires. Face validity refers to whether the questions in a questionnaire appear to address the subject of interest – how does it look at face value? Content validity refers to how well the questionnaire measures what it is meant to measure – does it cover all aspects of the topic or concept it was designed to ask about? There are also other types of validity that questionnaires can be tested for, and each tells you about a different aspect of accuracy of the questionnaire. Reliability is different to validity: it is about the consistency of a measure – whether it measures the same thing when completed by different people and/or at different time points. Again, there are different types of reliability that questionnaires can be tested for.

The key message here is that in any study using a questionnaire, look for information on how the questionnaire was designed and whether it was tested and piloted. Researchers often state that a questionnaire has been used or tested before in another study, in a similar sample and/or setting. Questionnaires that have been formally tested before are usually referred to as validated (or pre-validated). The results of the testing and piloting should tell you whether the questionnaire is valid, i.e. that it elicits the information it seeks to obtain. It should also tell you whether it is reliable, i.e. that it can be understood in the same way, by each participant, at different points in time. Another advantage of using pre-existing questionnaires is that there should be published data from that questionnaire that can sometimes be used to compare with the new findings from it: authors often report on this in their discussion sections. Some surveys use a combination of pre-existing validated questionnaires and new questions designed for their specific needs. If the questionnaire (or questions) was not validated but was developed by the researchers themselves, and you cannot find evidence that they have undertaken a rigorous process to develop and pilot it, then keep this in mind when reading the rest of the paper.

Perry et al. (2015) used a number of pre-existing, validated questionnaires in their survey. They asked a broad range of questions relating to the mental health of their participants. Seeking data on a broader range of issues than just the mental health of nurses, which was the focus of the paper, the researchers sought information on the participants' knowledge of health promotion, lifestyle and behavioural interventions. They identified pre-existing, validated questionnaires to measure general health and risk of eating disorders. As they were validated, we can be confident that the questionnaires are robust. However, the administration of more than one questionnaire, or even one long questionnaire, does risk participant fatigue or participant burden which might lead to the questionnaires not being (fully) completed or even returned.

It is important to look at the response rate achieved by a survey and consider whether the length and complexity of the survey (the number and type of questions) might have been a factor in determining it. Perry et al. (2015) had a response rate of 31%. We will discuss the implications of this later in the chapter.

What might the questions in a survey look like?

Questions in a survey can be presented in different formats. They can be open or closed, they can ask you to rate your response to a statement, they can be multiple choice, or can invite you to provide a free text answer using your own words. The way the question is structured should depend on what the researcher is trying to find out. For example, some questions are clearly answerable by a yes or no answer: these are closed questions. For other questions, more detailed responses are required: they can have a list of pre-identified responses to choose from or they might be designed to enable the participant to provide an unprompted, free text response. Some examples are given in Table 2.1.

Table 2.1   Different types of questions commonly found in a questionnaire

Question type	What this means	Example
Open ended	The way the question is written means it cannot be answered with a yes/no response and is answered using the words of the respondent	How was your experience of your first placement?
Closed ended	The way the question is written controls the format of the answer – the options for the answers are usually provided to choose from and it is often a one-word or short phrase answer	Did you enjoy your placement? Yes/No
Multiple response questions	This is a closed question that offers several different answers to choose from – and allows the respondent to select more than one	What was good about your placement? Tick all that apply: • Good learning environment • Supportive staff • Convenient location • Challenging • Pleasant environment • Support from university • Other, specify:

Question type	What this means	Example
Rating questions	These ask respondents to rate things (such as level of satisfaction) using a common scale	How would you rate your placement on a scale of 1-10 (where 1 is bad and 10 is good)?
Likert scale	These are typically a five (or seven) point scale which allows the respondent to express how much they agree or disagree with a statement	I enjoyed my placement: Strongly agree/agree/neither agree nor disagree/disagree/ strongly disagree
Free text	This is typically an invitation to the respondent to provide any other information or thoughts they would like to at the end of a questionnaire or survey - or they are included within the questionnaire to allow the respondent to specify or clarify an answer	Is there anything else you would like to tell us about your placement?

Perry et al. (2015) asked their participants to complete a combination of pre-existing questionnaires, which are likely to have included different types of questions from the examples above.

Is the survey itself made available to the reader?

When you read a paper about a survey, it is much easier to make sense of it if you have access to the actual survey or questionnaire used. If it is a pre-existing questionnaire, then you might be able to access this online or via the reference provided in the paper. If the questionnaire is not pre-existing, then, whilst you might be able to infer some of the questions from the results provided, you can only gain a clear picture of the survey if you can see the actual questions or questionnaire that was used. The reason for this is that you can see what questions were asked, what topics were covered, how they were asked and the order of the questions: each of these may impact on the answers given. However, the questionnaire is often not included in a paper due to limitations in the word count in academic journals, although they can sometimes be provided as an online appendix to the paper, or supplement. When the questions are not included, you can try to obtain a copy of the questionnaire from the authors; there is usually one author who is identified as the 'corresponding author' on a paper for this sort of query. In Perry et al., we can't see the actual questions that were asked in the questionnaires, but they do provide references to the questionnaires they used – so we could go and look these up and check them out. What we do know is that respondents completed a wide selection of previously used questionnaires.

> **SURVEY INSTRUMENT**
>
> The survey tool was compiled of validated tools and questions. Family and medical history and health risk-related characteristics were sought using the formats employed by the Australian Longitudinal Study of Women's Health (ALSWH; see www.alswh.org.au) and the Health in Men Study (HIMS; see www.wacha.org.au/hims.html), including current psycho-active medications, tobacco and alcohol use.

Who did they send the survey to?

Once you have established your confidence in the survey instrument itself (the questions/questionnaire(s) used), the next thing to consider is who it was distributed to – in other words, who was in the sample? The concept of a sample was discussed in Chapter 1. In an ideal world, we would send a survey to, and receive responses from, everyone in a population and we would then be confident that we had the full range of answers. Clearly, this is not possible. Instead, researchers identify a sample of people with whom they will undertake their research. The generalisability of the findings from the sample to the wider population must therefore always be considered.

So, ideally, the sample will be representative of the total population in which you are interested. It is the task of researchers to identify how this might best be achieved. For example, a questionnaire undertaken on a sample of nurses identified from those going in and out of the hospital library late in the evening and asked their views on the hospital's general working conditions may not represent the entire nursing population's views on this, whereas the views of a sample of nurses obtained at random from the hospital payroll should be more representative. Similarly, if the survey was being conducted in a number of hospitals, we would want to check that a range of different types of hospitals had been included in the sample; for example, community hospitals in addition to referral centres. So, depending on the question the study is addressing, we may need to check how the sampling was done at more than one level: the individual level (in this case, which nurses were approached) and the setting level (what type of hospitals they were from).

Perry et al. (2015) took their sample from nurses at two tertiary referral hospitals in one city in Australia. We can consider how representative the sample is to other hospitals such as non-tertiary referral centres, other hospitals in Australia and further afield; that is, whether it is reasonable to generalise responses obtained from nurses at the tertiary referral hospitals to nurses at other hospitals in Australia or further afield.

How did they distribute the survey?

There are different ways to distribute a survey – none is perfect. You have probably experienced some of these yourself, such as online, by telephone or text message, or postally – or you may have been asked to answer some questions in person on the street or in a waiting room. Ideally, in order to get a full range of responses from a representative group of people, everyone who is offered or receives the survey would respond; that is, you would get answers to your questions from everyone in your sample. This is, of course, very rarely achieved. Every method of distribution has its drawbacks, and it can be difficult to get a good response rate: the response rate is the number of completed surveys compared to the number distributed, and it is almost impossible to get a response rate of 100%. This means that most, if not all, research undertaken using surveys is subject to respondent bias; not everyone returns the survey and those who do return it might be different to those who do not (and so may give different answers), resulting in a non-representative sample.

How the survey is distributed can impact on the response rate. Studies have even been done on the effects of different distribution strategies on response rates; for example, whether providing a freepost, pre-franked envelope on a postal survey achieves a different response rate to using envelopes with stamps physically stuck on. Either way, in a postal survey, those responding need to be able to access a postbox! So, this method may not work so well for those who might have difficulty with this. Different distribution and return methods also have cost implications for the study overall, so that may have been a factor in why the researchers chose a particular method. Internet surveys might seem to solve these problems, but – as with post-boxes – they do restrict the sample to those who have access to the technology. It can also be difficult to know exactly who the sample is as e-questionnaires can easily be forwarded. The distribution and return of surveys are clearly a major challenge and one which has a major impact on the findings. It is therefore important to look for this detail in the paper and think about how such things might impact on the survey's findings. It is unlikely you will know anything about the people who didn't respond, and it is never possible to know what those who didn't respond would have told us. Furthermore, even for those who do respond, they do not always complete the survey in full, limiting the usefulness of the data collected by the survey.

Perry et al. (2015) distributed their survey to nurses via the hospitals' internal post. They sent their survey to 1,215 nurses and received 381 surveys back: a 31.4% response rate. Distribution via the internal post would mean that only those currently in work, and not those off sick due to their mental health, for example, would receive it. The researchers also noted that not all of the questionnaires within the survey were fully completed.

RESULTS

A total of 1,215 surveys were distributed with a usable response rate of 381 (31.4%).

This 31% response rate might seem low, but this is actually fairly normal (if not quite good) for a postal survey (Sinclair et al., 2012). This demonstrates the potential limitations of a survey approach. If less than a third of the nurses returned the surveys, it means there is no data on the views of more than two-thirds of the nurses (those who did not return them), and, for many reasons, there might be something different about those who returned the survey and those who did not. Those who returned the survey might have been exceptionally compliant, resilient or hard-working, or may have held another characteristic that could impact on the answers they gave, but it is not possible to tell. In other words, a major limitation of a survey is that we are unlikely to get a 100% response rate, and this means that we do not collect data from everyone in the sample and this can lead to bias in the results and conclusions that can be drawn.

Researchers can offer incentives such as a reward or an entry into a prize draw for completion of a survey, or they can advertise the survey in multiple ways to encourage responses – for example, by putting posters up about a survey to raise its profile and encourage its completion and return – but there is little a researcher can do about a low response rate, once it has occurred, beyond sending potential participants reminders. Perry et al. (2015) sent a reminder by email: they stated that the survey was anonymous, so it is likely that the email reminder went to everybody in the sample rather than targeting those who had not responded. Another option is to consider changing the method of distribution and return of the survey to try and increase the likelihood of returns. For example, Perry et al. (2015) might have considered distributing the questionnaires at the entrance of the hospital, providing opportunities for staff to complete them on the spot or providing highly visible boxes for their return, but this physical presence would have been time-consuming and therefore costly in terms of resources. It might also have reduced the anonymity of the survey or even been seen as coercive; nurses might have felt they had no option but to complete the survey and that there may be implications if they did not, which (as well as raising questions of ethics) could affect their responses.

So, researchers are dependent on the motivation of the would-be participant to complete and return surveys – although this is true of most study methods. You can see why, for some government surveys, completion is compulsory and non-completion can result in a penalty. Such sanctions are not appropriate for health care researchers; indeed, researchers are generally ethically obliged to inform would-be participants that participation in terms of the completion and return of the survey is entirely voluntary, that there is no obligation to do so and that, if they are patients, their decision to take part or not will not impact on their care.

How did they analyse the results?

In a small survey, it is possible to read through participants' answers and add up, tally or tabulate the responses by hand. When lecturers ask a small group of students to evaluate their teaching in a short survey, their responses are typically analysed by hand without the need to use a computer to assist in the analysis. In a larger survey, such as Perry et al. (2015), this is not possible. Perry et al. (2015) used an extensive set of questionnaires and these were distributed to over 1000 nurses. Even with a low response rate, this will generate a large amount of data. For surveys such as these, responses are typically entered into a database which helps to manage the large amount of data and the analysis.

Answers to questions that are not already numbers are typically converted into numerical responses for entry into the database, spreadsheet or statistical software. For example, a 'yes' response might be given a score of 1 and a 'no' response scored either 0 or 2; the actual numbers themselves don't really matter, what is important is that each type of answer is given a distinct number. This is sometimes called coding. The data entered are then relatively easy to analyse within the database, spreadsheet or statistical software program (such as SPSS or Minitab): Perry et al (2015) used SPSS. Such programs will collate all the responses to the questions across the respondents (the sample) and can then summarise and analyse the responses. Free text responses are sometimes numerically coded like this but will more often be analysed separately, as text.

DATA ANALYSES

Data were entered and analysed using the Statistical Package for the Social Sciences (SPSS) for Windows Version 21. Descriptive analyses used means and standard deviations, frequency and percentage according to the level of the variable. The independent predictors of mental health and vitality (both composite scores of the relevant SF-36 domains) were determined using linear regression analyses. For both models forced entry was used of potentially explanatory…

Analysis of numerical data from a survey is generally both descriptive and inferential. In this book, we are focusing on helping you to understand the results in a paper rather than explaining the statistical methods involved. Descriptive analysis simply describes what is in the data collected (e.g. the number of participants in different age groups), whilst inferential analysis enables researchers to make generalisations to the wider population. We can also interpret the data which helps us make sense of the data that has been collected, analysed and presented. Perry et al. (2015) report descriptive data in their paper. For example, they tell us the number of respondents who reported a mental health condition:

MENTAL HEALTH

Altogether 53 nurses (13.9%) reported a history of diagnosed mental health disorders with n = 49 (12.9) listing anxiety/depression; 22 (5.8%) were currently taking a psychoactive medication. One-fifth (n = 80, 21%) reported disordered eating behaviours …

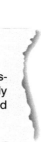

These are a straight report of the results that the reader could similarly have gleaned had they had access to all of the survey's responses. However, in order to help the reader, there are different ways that descriptive statistics can be presented. You will often see the mean, median, mode and standard deviation of the results presented in a paper. Table 2.2 gives you standard definitions of some of these.

Table 2.2   Definitions of commonly used descriptive statistical terms

Mean	Calculated by adding up all the numbers relating to a question (e.g. the ages of respondents) and dividing by the number of values in the dataset (e.g. the number of survey respondents)
Median	The middle value of the dataset where the values are ordered from smallest to greatest, e.g. youngest to oldest - the age right in the middle will be the median
Mode	The number that occurs most frequently in the dataset, e.g. the most common age reported
Range	The maximum value minus the minimum datapoint, e.g. in Perry's study, the range was 47 years, as the oldest participant (the maximum age) was 67 years, and the youngest (the minimum age) 20 years
Standard deviation	This describes how much the data value deviates from the mean: a high standard deviation means that, in general, the data is spread across a wider range of values (and is therefore further) from the mean; the lower it is, the more the data is clustered around the mean.

In the paper's text, Perry et al. (2015) gave the mean age of their sample as 39.9 years and the proportion of people over 40 and 50 years of age. And if you look at Table 1 in the paper, Perry et al. also give the standard deviation.

The authors also interpreted their results. This is where the results from one question are compared with the results from other questions or are compared for different sub-samples (smaller groups of interest within the sample) so that patterns in the data can be identified. For example, Perry et al. (2015) analysed whether those who smoked had better or worse mental health than those who did not, and whether those who lived alone had better or worse mental health than those who did not. They also determined the independent predictors of mental health and vitality using linear regression: a statistical test used to determine the association between different variables with an identified outcome variable, whilst also taking into account any associations across variables. This form of analysis allows for consideration of the effects across variables, such as, for example, whether differences in alcohol drinking and smoking patterns between those living alone or with others are associated with differences in mental health. In other words, they pulled together the results from the questionnaires and looked for patterns of association between the characteristics described in the data and the mental health of those who completed the survey.

Perry et al. (2015) also used inferential statistics in order to generalise from the sample of nurses included in the study to the wider population of nurses. Researchers can, for example, predict – using appropriate statistical tests – whether the findings from a study can be applied to the wider population, and the confidence they have in making these predictions. The type of numerical analysis conducted will depend both on the research question (what it was the researchers wanted to find out) and the type of data collected.

Perry et al. (2015) calculated confidence intervals in order to make generalisations. Confidence intervals reflect the confidence (or certainty) we can have that the results found in a sample are an accurate indication of the true population prevalence: they give numerical limits to a 'common-sense' approach. Confidence intervals estimate the confidence or certainty that the sample reflects a range within which the true score is known to lie. The smaller the interval or range of the confidence intervals, the more confident you can be that the results in the study reflect the results you would find in the larger population. Using a formula, the confidence intervals – upper and lower – are calculated. Confidence levels are slightly different to the intervals: a 95 per cent confidence level means that we can be 95 per cent confident that the true population prevalence lies between the lower and upper confidence interval, but there is a 5% chance that the finding was simply a result of chance. So, confidence intervals predict the confidence or margin of error we have in the findings of a study; the smaller the confidence intervals, the more confident the researchers are in the findings' generalisability.

BOX 2.1: AN EXAMPLE OF A CONFIDENCE INTERVAL CALCULATION

100 students are asked to document the number of hours per week spent using a mobile phone. The mean number of hours is 4. The confidence intervals are calculated as 2.5–5.6. This means that you can be 95 per cent confident that students spend between 2.5 and 5.6 hours per week using a mobile phone.

Rather than explain how to do these tests, our aim here is to help you understand what they mean so you can understand a paper better when you read it. Suggested further reading on the use of statistics in research is given at the end of this chapter.

At the end of a survey, there is often a free text section where participants can add their own unstructured responses – perhaps explaining why they gave the answer they did to a particular question or providing some additional information they think might be relevant. It is hard to convert these sorts of answers into numbers and enter them into a database to analyse them, so researchers often need to take a different approach. They need to read and understand the range of answers given and, if appropriate, group them meaningfully in order to summarise and report them. Perry et al. (2015) do not report any free text data; all their analysis was numerical.

How did they present the results?

It is good practice to start the results section of a survey paper by reporting the response rate and the characteristics of those who responded (and, if possible, comparing them to those who did not). This helps us to judge how representative those who responded are of the whole sample, and of the population from which the sample was drawn. It can also help you consider how representative they are of the population in your own setting, especially if you are considering using the findings of the survey to change your clinical practice. For example, Perry et al. (2015) report the number of people who completed the questionnaire and provide some demographic details about the sample in Table 1 of the paper (see Figure 2.1).

Table 1 **Socio-demographic and work characteristics**

From: The mental health of nurses in acute teaching hospital settings: a cross-sectional survey

Characteristic (n = 381)	Mean	SD
Age (range 20–67) years	39.9	11.7
	n	%
Female	315	82.7
Lives alone	96	25.2
Country of birth (n = 372)		
Australia	170	45.7
United Kingdom or Ireland	70	18.2
Asia	65	17.5
Europe	30	8.1
Other	39	10.5
Work classification		
*RN	216	56.7
*CNS/CNC/NP	84	22.1
*NM/NUM/Manager	41	10.7
*EN	18	4.7
*CNE/Educator	18	4.7
Other	4	1.1
Work contract		
Full time	303	79.6
Part-time (<1 FTE)	65	17.2
Casual/agency	12	3.2
Highest qualification		
Bachelor degree	160	42.0
Post-graduate certificate/diploma	84	22.0
Masters degree/ doctorate	56	14.7
Certificate only	41	10.8
Diploma only	36	9.5

*Registered Nurse/Clinical Nurse Specialist/Clinical Nurse Consultant/Nurse Practitioner/Nurse Manager/Nursing Unit Manager/Enrolled Nurse/Clinical Nurse Educator.

Figure 2.1   Table 1 from Perry et al. (2015)

Note that when the sample is reported in Table 1 of the paper, both the number of people and the percentage of people are given. It is good practice to state the number of participants (often referred to as 'n = ') in addition to the percentage of participants (%), as percentages alone can be misleading. For example, saying that 30% of 100,000 people agree with something might have very different implications to 30% of just 10 people. The researchers also present the mean (average) for the sample's characteristics and the standard deviation (the measure of distribution in the sample, as described above).

Perry et al. (2015) present their results using a combination of narrative text, in which words are used to report the main findings, and accompanying tables, that present the complete findings numerically. The results of the questionnaire describe the number of nurses who had experienced mental health disorders and the factors associated with this. For example, Table 2 in the paper (shown in Figure 2.2) presents the responses to individual questions about mental health and symptoms that might be associated with mental health, such as sleeping patterns.

Table 2 **Symptoms potentially related to mental health issues experienced sometimes or often in last 12 months; whether help sought**

From: The mental health of nurses in acute teaching hospital settings: a cross-sectional survey

	Sometimes		Often		Sought help	
	n	%	n	%	n	%
Headaches	101	26.5	38	10.0	29	7.6
Severe tiredness	100	26.2	39	10.2	22	5.8
Indigestion/heartburn	50	13.1	15	3.9	22	5.8
Anxiety	45	11.8	12	3.1	22	5.8
Night sweats	27	7.1	19	5.0	13	3.4
Depression	29	7.6	12	3.1	24	6.3
Palpitations	31	8.1	4	1.0	2	0.5
Sleep problems (current)						
Waking in the early hours	212	55.6				
Sleeping badly at night	128	33.6				
Taking a long time to get to sleep	116	30.4				
Worrying keeping you awake at night	102	26.8				
Lying awake most of the night	70	18.4				
Sleep problems score ≥ 1 (0–5)	268	70.3				
Eating disorders score ≥ 2 (0–5)	80	20.9				

Figure 2.2   Table 2 from Perry et al. (2015)

Perry et al. (2015) then present the results of an analysis of the link between the respondents' self-reported mental health and the symptoms identified. So, in this section of the results, you can see that the researchers have moved beyond the descriptive (Tables 1–3 in the paper) towards being more interpretative – calculating possible relationships between the variables using a statistical test referred to as linear regression (Table 4 in the paper). For example, they reported that nurses had better mental health if they had better physical health. Table 4 in the paper (shown in Figure 2.3) reports the confidence intervals for some of the data; that is, how generalisable the findings are to the wider population.

Table 4 **Predictors of mental health (SF36 Mental composite scale)**

From: The mental health of nurses in acute teaching hospital settings: a cross-sectional survey

Characteristics	Beta	95% confidence interval	P value
General health	3.17	2.68 – 6.15	<0.001
Live alone versus with partner	7.35	9.6 – 5.4	<0.001
Total sum of symptoms	-2.06	-4.0 – -0.3	0.001
Sleep problems, total	-1.36	-2.91 – -0.86	0.006
Disordered eating	-2.00	-3.29 – -0.48	0.006
Informal carer role	-5.59	-7.24 – -3.1	0.025
Night shifts	-3.04	-2.53 – -5.54	0.04

Model statistics r^2 = .340, f = 8.784, p <0.001.

Figure 2.3   Table 4 from Perry et al. (2015)

On its own, Table 4 (Figure 2.3) may be difficult to understand, but the narrative explanation Perry et al. provide helps to grasp it.

Predictors (Table 4). Nurses had better mental health if they had better general health (β = 4.14); if they lived with a spouse or partner rather than alone (β = 7.35) or were not an informal carer (β = –5.59); if they had fewer symptoms (β = –0.206), sleep problems (β = –1.36) or disordered eating behaviours (β = –2.00); if they did not work nights (β = 3.04).

At this point, you can see why the accurate, meaningful and representative collection of data is so important. Calculating precise statistics about the numerical relationship between different variables is only a meaningful activity if a representative sample of people completed and returned the survey and completed those surveys in full. Perry et al. (2015) obtained a response rate of 31%, meaning that the results may not be generalisable to the wider population, even if the confidence intervals indicate some precision in the findings.

Was the study ethical?

In Chapter 1, we explained that the main ethical considerations a reader of a study should be aware of are the risk of harm to the participants and a consideration of informed consent. Both of these are relevant to this study. Perry et al. (2015) included a section dedicated to ethical considerations, stating that ethical approval was in place. When reading a study, you might feel that the approach used to contact people to invite them to take part (or to send reminders about responding) was intrusive, even though it was approved by ethical review. In Perry et al. (2015), the return of the survey was considered an indication of consent to take part. In most studies, those who agree to take part are usually asked to sign a consent form, but with a survey sometimes just its return, completed, is taken as consent to take part.

DATA COLLECTION

Letters of invitation, Information Statements and copies of the survey were delivered and returned through the internal hospital post; reminders were delivered by email. Return of a completed survey was understood to convey consent to participate in this study. Data were collected over four months in 2011–2012 at the two sites.

The return of the survey does not generally tell us about any harm that might have occurred, unless a participant specifically mentions this in the return (perhaps in a free text comments box at the end of the questionnaire). The risk of the survey triggering unpleasant memories is real; questioning staff about their mental health could cause unintended harm to participants, despite the good intention of the study. It is unknown whether any participants suffered additional mental health problems as a result of taking part in this survey. One way to ascertain this might be to review uptake of any support that may have been offered to participants who experienced problems as a result of taking part, or to undertake a follow-on study to explore the effects of taking part in a study that might trigger negative or challenging memories. In Perry et al. (2015), it was assumed that participants would contact their general practitioner should untoward adverse effects arise from receiving or taking part in the survey – it would therefore not be possible to monitor and report on this unless participants were followed up afterwards.

How confident can we be of the results?

The results obtained from a survey are relevant to those who took part in the survey; however, in quantitative research, we are interested in how generalisable these results might be to the wider population. For most quantitative research – surveys included – the goal is to find out information from a sample of people and to be able to generalise this to the wider population it is meant to represent. So, in the case of Perry et al. (2015), it is important to discuss the extent to which the survey sheds light on the mental health of nurses more generally.

We have identified some of the main limitations of survey research. You might be wondering if generalising to the wider population is at all possible given the pitfalls we have described. Perry et al. (2015) found a high level of mental health concerns in their study, both diagnosed as mental health problems and noted as symptoms that might indicate the presence of mental health issues. Yet, the response rate does not indicate that those who responded are representative of the wider population; we will never know how those who did not respond would have responded. It could be that those with an interest and concern in their own mental health were more likely to respond to the survey but, as we do not know about those who did not respond, this is not possible to say. This is why it is important to identify and understand who the sample were, when and how they were contacted, and how many of the people in the sample returned the survey and returned it fully completed.

It is good practice for researchers to consider and reflect on this in the discussion section of their papers. This should happen in two ways – first, the authors compare their findings to those of other, relevant research (to put it in context) and, second, the authors write a paragraph about the strengths and limitations of their study. Perry et al. (2015) do this in a section headed 'Limitations'.

LIMITATIONS

Study limitations include the response rate; whilst 31.4% was acceptable for a general survey, results should be interpreted with caution. It is possible that those positively inclined towards health issues participated in the study and were attitudinally and/or behaviourally different to those who chose not to participate.

In summary

In this chapter we have explored what you should be looking for when you read a survey or a questionnaire-based study. Designing a valid and reliable survey is tricky. Once carefully designed and tested (piloted), it then needs to be distributed to a representative sample of people in a way that is most likely to achieve a good response rate from them. We need to know that the survey is valid and reliable, and is returned by a representative group of people contacted, rather than a particular subset. Without this, the information obtained from the survey may not be representative, and generalisation to the wider population may be difficult. These conditions are not easy to achieve, and this is why, despite appearing simple, surveys have limitations and are often not considered strong forms of evidence. However, they are often the only practical way to obtain data and, as the Perry et al. (2015) study indicates, they can produce useful findings which would otherwise not be evident.

BOX 2.2: QUESTIONS TO ASK YOURSELF ABOUT A SURVEY

When reading a survey paper, always ask:

- How was the survey designed?
- How was it distributed?
- Who was in the sample?
- How many people (and who) responded?
- Does the analysis make sense?
- Are the conclusions based on the results?

REFLECTIONS FROM ONE OF THE PAPER'S AUTHORS

We were able to make contact with Lin Perry, the lead author of this paper. Lin provided very generous feedback on a draft of this chapter, which we have summarised here:

Readers will appreciate the importance of this topic – the 'emotional labour' of nursing is well recognised within the profession at both personal and workforce levels. However, surprisingly little attention has been focused on understanding the health, including mental health, of this workforce. This survey, of which this paper reports the mental health components, was the preparatory and 'pilot' stage for a larger, nationally representative study, although the journal's reviewers felt the sample size was too large for us to use the term 'pilot'.

The importance of the response rate is a good point, against which we had to balance the importance for this survey of anonymity of response and the risk of perceived coercion from research team members in senior hospital positions. We considered sending the survey via email as an online link; however, the experience of previous surveys at these sites indicated that the previously noted limited access of registered nurses, particularly, to personal computers at work rendered this a restrictive approach likely to yield low response rates.

SUGGESTED READING

Harris, M. and Taylor, G. (2020) *Medical Statistics Made Easy*. Banbury: Scion Publishing.
Oppenheim, A. N. (1992) *Questionnaire, Design, Interviewing and Attitude Measurement*. London: Pinter.

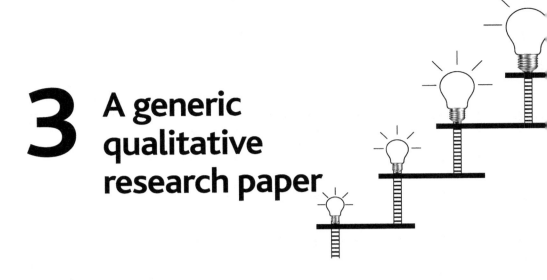

3 A generic qualitative research paper

What is qualitative research?

When we want to know about something, we often go and speak to someone. If that conversation is with a key person and becomes in-depth, it can really help us gain an insight into the thing we are interested in. As we talk, and our understanding grows, we ask questions when we are not sure about something the person has said, or where we want to know more, and so gain a deeper insight into the topic. In many ways, this is the basis of qualitative research. Instead of seeking the opinion of hundreds of people about pre-specified questions, for example through a survey, qualitative research allows us to explore an area in greater depth, often through in-depth interviews with people who have experience of what we are interested in, so that we can gain a greater understanding. Qualitative research is often considered to be an umbrella term to describe a research approach made up of a range of exploratory methods, some of which we discuss in later chapters of this book. The term 'qualitative research' can also be used to describe a method in its own right.

The qualitative paper we will explore in this chapter is:

Borglin, G., Rathel, K., Paulsson, H. and Sjogren Forss, K. (2020) Registered nurses' (RNs) experiences of managing depressive symptoms at care centres for older people: A qualitative descriptive study. *BMC Nursing*, 18: article no. 43.

In this study, the researchers sought to gain an understanding of the ways in which nurses manage the common symptoms of depression in the people they look after. This is an important area of care, and the study aimed to understand how these symptoms might be addressed and better managed in future care provision.

Get yourself a copy of the paper, read it through, then read through the rest of the chapter, finding the points we identify in the paper: https://bmcnurs.biomedcentral.com/articles/10.1186/s12912-019-0368-5

Scan the QR code to be taken straight to the paper.

What does the abstract and information about the authors tell me?

In Chapter 2, we introduced you to the important features of an abstract. The abstract should be a concise account of the study that provides enough information to enable you to assess whether to access the paper in full.

In their abstract, Borglin et al. (2020) give a concise summary of their study. It is clear from the background section of the abstract what the rationale was for the study. The methods are summarised and the headline results are clearly presented. The researchers were interested in understanding nurses' experiences of identifying and intervening in cases of depressive symptoms in older people in a particular care setting; they wanted to increase understanding of this important topic. They conducted a qualitative descriptive study to achieve this.

ABSTRACT

Background

Depressive symptoms and/or depression are commonly experienced by older people. Both are underdiagnosed, undertreated and regularly overlooked by health care professionals. Health care facilities for people aged ≥75 years have been in place in Sweden since 2015. The aim of these care centres, which are managed by registered nurses (RNs), is to offer care adjusted to cater to the complex needs and health problems of older people. Although the mental health of older people is prioritised in these centres, research into the experience of RNs of depressive symptoms and/or depression in older people in this setting is limited. Therefore, this study aimed to illuminate RNs', working at care centres for older people, experience of identifying and intervening in cases of depressive symptoms.

Methods

The data for this qualitative descriptive study were collected through interviews ($n = 10$) with RNs working at 10 care centres for older people in southern Sweden. The transcribed texts were analysed using inductive content analysis.

Results

The participants' experiences could be understood through four predominant themes: (1) challenging to identify, (2) described interventions, (3) prerequisites for identification, and (4) contextual influences. Key findings were that it was difficult to identify depression as it often manifested as physical symptoms; evidence-based nursing interventions were generally not the first-line treatment used; trust, continuity and the ability of RNs to think laterally and the context influenced the ability of RNs to manage older people's depressive symptoms and/or depression.

Conclusions

The process of identifying depressive symptoms and performing an appropriate intervention was found to be complex, especially as older people were reluctant to present at the centres and provided obscure reasons for doing so. A nurse–patient relationship that was built on trust and was characterised by continuity of care was identified as a necessary prerequisite. Appropriate nursing interventions – afforded the same status as pharmacological treatment – are warranted as the first-line treatment of depression. Further research is also needed into efficacious nursing interventions targeting depressive symptoms and/or depression.

Keywords: Care centres for older people, Content analysis, Nursing, Qualitative research, Registered nurses

Looking at who the authors are also tells you something about the study; always consider carefully who they are and where they are from. In this paper, the authors are nurse academics at the University of Oslo in Norway and the University of Malmo in Sweden, where they are part of a nursing institution in which research into care of the elderly is an important component. This is evident by the numbers of related publications which are listed under the author names on the institution's website. This suggests that this is an area of special interest for these authors and evidence of an established track record in this field.

Is there a clear research question or aim addressed by the research?

All research papers should have a clear research question or aim. This might be different from the title of a research paper. For example, the title of this paper is a statement: *Registered nurses' experiences of managing depressive symptoms at care centres for older people: A qualitative descriptive study*. You should look for an explicit question or aim that tells you the exact focus of the research.

Further on in the paper, the authors state their specific aim, which is: 'to illuminate RNs', working at CCOPs (care centres for older people), experience of identifying and intervening in cases of depressive symptoms among older people'. Do note that the aim or research question does not always come after a sub-heading (so it may not be labelled) but can sometimes be found at the end of the introduction – as in this case – or at the beginning of the methods. What is important is that you can recognise a clear research question or aim for the study in the paper.

To our knowledge, this is one of the first studies exploring this. Thus, this study aimed to illuminate RNs', working at CCOPs, experience of identifying and intervening in cases of depressive symptoms among older people.

In this study, the aim is broken down into two aspects of managing depressive symptoms: how nurses identify symptoms of depression and the interventions for them. It is important to note that there is no hypothesis in a qualitative study: the research is exploratory. Researchers are not setting out to prove or disprove an idea but are aiming to develop our understanding of a topic through the collection of in-depth, rich data.

How was the study designed?

This research study is qualitative. There are many different qualitative research designs. You may be familiar with the names of some of the different designs which include grounded theory, ethnography and phenomenology. We will explore some of these specific qualitative research designs in other chapters of this book. However, like many authors, Borglin et al. (2020) did not align their qualitative study to a specific design but instead described the study as a 'qualitative descriptive study'. Some readers who have studied research methods previously might be surprised by the simplicity of this and may be tempted to conclude that a qualitative study without a named design is not a 'proper' qualitative study. The research methods literature relating to qualitative designs would not support this view. There are lots of different qualitative research designs. Some research studies state alignment to a design but do not then utilise this in any detail, whilst other studies suggest that they have some but not full alignment to a particular design or method. Although the varying designs tend to be aligned with particular types of research question or aim, it is certainly not the established school of thought that all qualitative research must adhere to a named design.

This study is simply referred to as a qualitative descriptive study. This fits with the aim of the paper which is to illuminate the experiences of nurses in the way in which they identify and intervene in cases of depression – the term 'illuminate' suggests exploration and a desire to increase understanding. Qualitative research aims to explore, describe and understand phenomena in an in-depth and detailed way: in this case, the way in which nurses manage – through identification and intervention – depressive symptoms in older people in care centres. It does not intend to find out if one intervention works better than another. The researchers are not looking at what nursing interventions might be *effective* in managing depression – that would be a different research question requiring a different approach and research design or method and one that we will consider when we look at randomised controlled trials. Neither are they looking at the *causes* of depression – that would be another, different, research question requiring another different design and method, and one that we will be discussing when we look at cohort and case-control studies. Instead, the authors aimed to explore a phenomenon in-depth in order to describe and understand it.

In view of this, Borglin et al. (2020) designed a qualitative descriptive study, with the aim of understanding how nurses identify signs of depression in older people in that care setting, and what they do about it. The reason for doing this is concern that older people with depression might not have their symptoms recognised within that care setting. Exploring how nurses identify and intervene when patients show signs of depression – and maybe what they do not do – helps us consider how depression is managed within care settings for older people and whether more attention to the assessment and management of depression in those settings might lead to improved care.

When Borglin et al. (2020) designed their study, they needed to find a method that would allow them an in-depth exploration of the way in which nurses assessed the older people in their care. A questionnaire could get them some surface-level information but would not be able to illicit a more detailed, deeper understanding, for which more in-depth conversations with the nurses would be needed. Their choice of a qualitative approach and method was therefore appropriate for their aim.

What questions might be asked in a qualitative study?

The questions asked of participants in a qualitative study are generally open, and the interview schedule – the set of questions asked in the study – is usually unstructured or semi-structured. This means that the researcher has some flexibility in terms of what questions are asked, how they are asked and the order in which they are asked. This is useful as the purpose of the questions in a qualitative study is to generate an in-depth discussion that is not led or controlled by the interview schedule. Ideally, the discussion is led by the participant, and the role of the researcher is to keep the discussion on track – focused on the interview topic, whilst probing or prompting the participant to develop their ideas or give further detail on what they have shared in the interview. In a semi-structured interview, a set of questions may be prepared but there is some flexibility in how and when they are asked, whereas in an unstructured interview there may just be a list of topics to cover: in this case, the interview schedule is sometimes called a topic guide.

Borglin et al. (2020) used a very open, unstructured method – they stated that their interviews were based on one key question that focused on an episode of care in which the participant looked after a patient with depressive symptoms.

DATA COLLECTION

The data were collected through interviews [17]. The interviews were based on one key question: 'Can you please tell me about a situation in which you (as an RN at a CCOP) have been in contact with older people with depressive symptoms?' Probing, i.e. 'Can you please give me an example?' or 'Can you please tell me more?', was used, when necessary.

It is important to know where the topics or questions came from in a qualitative study and whether they were first piloted (which we explain below). In terms of where the topics or questions came from, we can check the paper for information to help us:

- Why were those topics covered, or questions asked? What was the rationale? For example, were the topic areas based on pre-existing evidence from other studies or identified as the result of a literature review?
- Were they identified through initial discussions with members of the public or patients who have experience or knowledge of the topic, or identified through discussions with relevant health care professionals?
- Were they informed by existing theories or other literature?

In terms of piloting, it can be useful to try out an interview schedule or topic guide with a very small number of people who are similar in a relevant way to those under study. This helps identify whether the topics or questions cover everything that they need to, or whether how the questions are asked is appropriate (or perhaps sensitive enough) given the study aims. Borglin et al. (2020) piloted their key question with two registered nurses at two different care centres to ensure relevance and understandability.

The key question was initially tested on two RNs at two different CCOPs, to ensure its relevance and understandability in relation to the study objective. As this did not lead to any changes, the data from the test interviews were included in the analysis.

Note that although these were pilot interviews, as they didn't result in any changes to the interview questions, Borglin et al. (2020) decided to keep and use these interviews as part of their dataset. If they had made significant changes to the questions as a result of these pilot interviews, then they would probably not have been included in the final dataset if the researcher felt the interview hadn't really worked.

Is the interview schedule or topic guide made available to the reader?

We have noted that qualitative interviews are generally guided by an interview schedule but, unlike a questionnaire, it is not the intention of the interviewer to keep to a script. The nature of qualitative interviews is that they will trigger conversations that cannot necessarily be predicted and should include open-ended, exploratory questions which will encourage the participant to discuss what is most pertinent to them in relation to the topic. However, as we noted in the chapter on surveys, when you read a paper it can be helpful if you can see the actual data collection tool – in this case, the interview schedule or topic guide. Sometimes this is described in the text or provided in a box within a paper, sometimes it is provided as an online supplement, but often it does not appear at all. As with surveys, whilst you might be able to infer some of the questions from the results, actually seeing what topics were asked about, and what were not, can be useful – although you won't know exactly how they were asked, or asked about, in each interview. In this study, there was only one main interview question, which we discussed earlier. This is made available to the reader.

Who was invited to participate in the study?

Qualitative research generally involves smaller sample sizes than quantitative research. The aim of qualitative research is not to generalise to a wider population but to generate understanding and insight within a focused area or population. Thus, a sample size that enables us to make generalisations is not needed. What is needed, however, is a sample that will illuminate the range of experiences and perceptions of those identified as being relevant to the study (Malterud et al., 2016). With this in mind, those invited to participate in the study must be appropriate for that purpose – that is, they should represent the range of experiences and perceptions of interest. In the case of Borglin et al.'s (2020) study, the participants needed to have experience of working in a 'care of the older person' setting. Only people with this experience were eligible to take part in the study. This type of sample is often referred to as a purposive sample. It can also be referred to as a convenience sample, which, as its name suggests, involves inviting those who can be identified conveniently, but such a sample must also be fit for purpose. Some qualitative studies take this a step further and seek a range of particular characteristics in their sample in order to achieve that range of views and experiences – for example, they might have sought out some participants who were newly qualified, some who had been qualified for a long time, some who were new to the care setting, some who were well established, some with a mental health qualification and some without. Another approach is snowball sampling, in which participants might suggest others who they know have the experience that the researchers are looking for. There can be an overlap between the methods of sampling; what is important is that the researchers are clear about who their sample was, how they identified them and why.

Borglin et al. (2020) identified a convenience sample of participants. They approached the managers of 37 care centres for older people in Sweden. After some follow-up, ten managers agreed in principle that their staff could be invited to take part in the study. We do not know how much these ten managers represented all the managers in the setting and whether those who did not respond might have led to the participation of nurses who might have had different perspectives. A total of ten nurses then participated in the study. This might seem a small sample, but the purpose of qualitative research is to achieve depth and a range of insight rather than to interview a large number of representative people (Malterud et al., 2016). Therefore, whether or not a sample of ten nurses is sufficient for this study depends on the depth of insight achieved in the interviews.

The researchers describe their sampling strategy as convenience. However, they also state that potential participants needed to have had one year's experience of working with older people and must currently be in that role; hence, the sampling strategy seems to contain aspects of a purposive sample. The requirement for experience of working with older people is referred to as an inclusion criterion. Inclusion criteria, as the name suggests, refer to the criteria required in participants in order to be eligible to participate. In this study, experience was a key inclusion criterion specific to the needs of this study; for a different question, the criteria might be based on gender, age or having had experience of a certain condition, for example. Studies may also state one or more exclusion criteria: criteria that, if present in a potential participant (who may meet all the inclusion criteria), will stop them from being included in the study.

In the paper, there is no detail given as to how the participants were identified once the managerial support for the study had been obtained. We are simply told that ten nurses agreed to take part. Information is not available about which care centres the participants came from or how potential participants were invited to participate. This will be discussed in the subsequent section on the ethics of the study.

Who undertook the interviews?

In a qualitative study, attention should be given to who undertook the interviews. Given the skill required to conduct qualitative interviews (due to their less structured nature), the quality of the interviews is, to some extent, dependent on the skills of the researcher. New researchers undertaking a project often comment that the later interviews in a set of interviews feel 'better' than the first few they conduct – this is often true for even very experienced researchers as skills and knowledge develop in relation to the topic area, and the participants, within a study. As with any study, qualitative or quantitative, the data collector (in this case, the interviewer) should be independent of the phenomenon or setting under study – so we would not expect to see a member of the care team, particularly a senior member, conducting the interviews as this could impact on the data collected. In any qualitative paper using interviews as a method, do take note of who did the interviewing as this could affect the quality of the data.

Borglin et al. (2020) reported that the interviews were conducted by either the second or third author of the paper. The affiliation of these authors brings a mix of academic and professional expertise to the project: one appears to be from an academic institution, the other from a care provider (although their job titles are not given). Information like this can sometimes be a bit hidden. In this paper, it was in the data collection section. We can see that the nurse interviews took between 30 and 50 minutes. In-depth interviews with patients are usually longer - lasting an hour or more.

> On average, they lasted between 30 and 50 min and were conducted by either the second or third author.

How did they analyse the results?

The analysis of qualitative interview data usually requires the transcription of audio-recorded interviews into text. This can become hundreds of pages of transcribed data for a small qualitative study which then need to be checked and anonymised before analysis formally begins. This interview data is then read closely, line by line, in order to identify common themes from the data – and there are different techniques for doing this.

In this study, interviews were transcribed (and analysed) by the team of researchers; often, professional transcription companies are used for the task of transcription. There are pros and cons to both ways of doing this: transcription by the team can start the analytic process but can be very time-consuming. Transcription by a professional company can be more efficient. Borglin et al. (2020) report undertaking an inductive content analysis. It is important to focus here on the term 'inductive'. The purpose of inductive data analysis is to infer a general understanding directly from the data collected, rather than to seek certain things from the data. That is, those analysing the data had no pre-conceived ideas about what they might find in the data: they did not approach the analysis of the interviews with a checklist of ideas or things to look for. Instead, they remained open-minded to the ideas expressed by the participants.

Content analysis is a method of analysing both qualitative and quantitative data. When qualitative data are analysed using content analysis, researchers are looking for content relevant to their question that is present across different interviews. This content is organised into categories and is essentially descriptive – it describes the phenomenon of interest. In their description of their analysis, Borglin et al. (2020) refer to the work of Elo and Kyngäs (2008) who describe the process of content analysis, incorporating the descriptive approach of identifying concepts and categories from data. However, Borglin et al. (2020) tell us that the interview data was coded and themes were developed – this suggests that they are using a thematic analysis rather than a content analysis. Thematic analysis is another method of qualitative data analysis. Instead of a reporting on content, a thematic analysis aims to identify themes which have an interpretative element rather than being descriptive. In practice, there is often a merging between these two approaches. It can be difficult for a researcher who is intending to undertake content analysis to remain purely descriptive rather than interpretative – and vice versa. In addition, it is also common for terms to be used interchangeably. This does not always make for easy understanding for the reader (Aveyard and Bradbury-Jones, 2019).

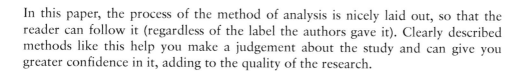

First, the transcribed material was read several times in order to ensure that the researcher was immersed in the data [18]. Second, key issues (i.e. meaning units) were condensed and coded manually using colouring pens. Third, the different coloured codes were then interpreted and compared for similarities and differences. Fourth, they were sorted into tentative subthemes, without losing their content [18]. In the initial part of the analysis, the second and third authors took the lead. However, all the authors separately read, analysed and discussed the text during the whole process to enhance the best possible account of the meaning found in the texts. Fifth and final, the authors agreed on 11 subthemes and four themes that unified the content within the subthemes formulated.

In this paper, the process of the method of analysis is nicely laid out, so that the reader can follow it (regardless of the label the authors gave it). Clearly described methods like this help you make a judgement about the study and can give you greater confidence in it, adding to the quality of the research.

How did they present the results?

In qualitative research, data are presented in the form of a narrative. There are very rarely numbers. There are no calculations, or statistical results reported – except for demographic details about participants. There is no hypothesis to prove or disprove. Data that has been collected from participants in a narrative and exploratory way is generally presented in this same way, albeit after an extensive process of analysis.

Borglin et al. (2020) present their results in the form of a narrative. The narrative is organised into themes which have been developed from the process of analysis described earlier. The purpose of the analysis is to summarise, interpret and explain the data gathered within the study. Therefore, in qualitative research, the presentation of findings is a substantial section of the paper which illuminates and addresses the study research question or aims. The themes are illustrated with supporting anonymised quotations from the interviews, providing evidence and examples of how the data from the interviews supports the analysis and links to the stated findings.

Not every quote can, or should, be included in a paper (just as we wouldn't include every individual piece of data from participants in a quantitative study), but the quotes should come from a range of the study participants rather than just one or two. Each quote should therefore have a participant identifier (usually a unique number, but sometimes a pseudonym) to help you judge this. This means that, although a clear audit trail of data cannot be provided, the clear inclusion of a range of quotes provides some evidence of how data from across the sample informed the developing themes:

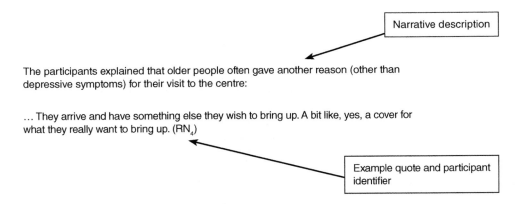

Narrative description

The participants explained that older people often gave another reason (other than depressive symptoms) for their visit to the centre:

… They arrive and have something else they wish to bring up. A bit like, yes, a cover for what they really want to bring up. (RN$_4$)

Example quote and participant identifier

In Borglin et al. (2020), four different themes with sub-themes outline the key findings of their study. These are illustrated in Table 1 of the paper, 'Examples of Process Analysis'. The themes are labelled as: the challenges to identifying depression, describing interventions for depression, prerequisites for managing depression, and other contextual influences. These themes and their sub-themes come directly from the data collected. They should also relate to the aim of the research so that data that is not relevant to the research question or aim is not reported. The themes and sub-themes are accompanied by a narrative or commentary which provides further context for the reader to understand the themes and data supporting them. However, in a content analysis, the grouping of data in the analysis is generally referred to as the creating of 'categories' rather than 'themes'. The term 'themes' generally implies an interpretative approach. Borglin et al. (2020) refer to their categories as themes. This illustrates how terms can be used interchangeably, as mentioned above (Aveyard and Bradbury-Jones, 2019). The analysis undertaken in the paper does seem to reflect a content analysis. However, later in the paper, the researchers mention an interpretative approach, illustrating the difficulties sometimes faced in clear alignment to either descriptive or interpretative methods in qualitative research.

Was the study ethical?

As we discussed in Chapter 2, it is always important to consider the ethics of any study, even if the study is published in a reputable, peer-reviewed journal. One ethical issue that is often very relevant to qualitative research is how participants are recruited. Interviews in qualitative research can sometimes ask participants to discuss personal, sensitive or intimate issues in a way that is often very different from completing a questionnaire. It is therefore important that participants do not feel obliged to participate in a qualitative (or any) study and that if the researchers have a connection with the organisation in which the potential participants work, then steps are taken to ensure that there is no direct connection between the researcher and those who might participate. So, for example, nurses who are invited to participate in a qualitative study that explores their satisfaction and intention to leave the organisation would rightly expect complete assurance that the researchers have no connection with the employing organisation and are certainly not senior members of staff working for that organisation.

Borglin et al. (2020) contacted many centres providing care for the older person and eventually obtained an agreement from ten organisations to participate. This does not mean that the organisations provided consent on behalf of their employees to participate. It merely means that the organisations were willing for their employees to be contacted and take part if they wanted to. We are not told in the paper how the potential participants within these agreeing organisations were approached, or by whom, and what measures were taken to ensure that staff did not feel any obligation to participate in the study. For example, if staff were informed about the study by their manager, they might feel an obligation to participate. Ideally, staff would have received information about the study, including an invitation to participate, with contact details of the researchers, so that those interested could get in touch with the research team and have any questions they had about the study answered. This information is not reported in the paper and so it is not clear how participants were informed about the study and invited to participate. The names of workplaces where participants were employed is rightly not included in the paper in order to prevent the identification of individuals.

At the end of the paper, we can see the authors state that the study had ethical approval and that informed consent was gained from participants.

ETHICS APPROVAL AND CONSENT TO PARTICIPATE

This study was conducted in compliance with the established ethical guidelines of the Declaration of Helsinki. Under the Swedish Ethical Review Act 2003:460 this study did not require ethical clearance, [but] we applied for and received ethical guidance from the Ethical Advisory Board in Southern Sweden. The researcher gave oral and written information and obtained written informed consent from all participants before the interviews. Participation was voluntary, and the participants had the right to withdraw at any time without further explanation. The participants gave consent for direct quotes from their interviews to be used in this paper. To ensure confidentiality, each quotation was assigned a pseudonym in the form of a number. Data were stored securely and anonymously in compliance with the Data Protection Act.

You will see that the authors state that participants gave informed consent for quotations from their interviews to be used in the paper. As we have noted, given that some workplaces employ only a few registered nurses, the name and location of the workplaces involved are not included in the paper to avoid the possibility of any individual being recognised. Whilst it states that participants can withdraw at any time, it is unclear whether any data they had already provided would then be excluded. Excluding data can be difficult in qualitative studies if data analysis has already commenced. Sometimes group interviews are used in qualitative studies, and this makes withdrawing actual data even more difficult. Potential participants therefore need to be informed of this before they consent to take part in a study. Borglin et al. (2020) also mention the data protection arrangements.

How confident can we be of the results of the study?

Every study has strengths and weaknesses which affect how confident we can be in the results and conclusions of the paper. In the previous chapter, we saw how this confidence can be achieved and expressed in numerical terms. For a qualitative study, there are no statistical tests to determine the precision of the findings. Instead, the confidence we can have depends on the transparency with which the study has been undertaken and reported, and on the explicit quality markers of the study. For qualitative research, there is no agreed definition of quality, making it hard for the reader: especially the inexperienced reader. Lincoln and Guba (1985) argue that the terms 'credibility', 'transferability', 'dependability' and 'confirmability' can be used to assess the quality of a qualitative study. They argue that all qualitative research should have a 'truth value' and that this can be determined by strategies that represent the hallmark of good qualitative research, such as keeping an accurate trail of the research process and transparency in the data analysis process. Borglin et al. (2020) provide a clear account of most of the steps they undertook for the study. It would be reasonable to assume that the findings are useful to all nurses working with older people in similar settings, but the extent to which the findings can be transferred to a wider population of nurses beyond these settings is unclear.

In summary

In this chapter we have summarised what you should look for when reading a generic (or general) qualitative research study. In this case, the qualitative research was not aligned to a particular qualitative design. Qualitative research can sometimes seem to be more straightforward and accessible than quantitative research as there are no hypotheses, no statistical analysis, and the findings are generally presented as a narrative. Yet undertaking qualitative research that is robust – that truly illuminates and explores a topic in-depth – is a complex activity. Sample sizes are generally (but appropriately) small and in-depth data is collected. These smaller sample sizes are appropriate as they allow a phenomenon to be explored in-depth. It is therefore important to consider whether this depth of understanding has been achieved and reported on in the paper, rather than simply a list of findings that could have been anticipated. Whilst the aim is not to generalise findings from qualitative research in the way that we might do from quantitative studies, researchers are seeking depth and breadth of understanding. Borglin et al.'s (2020) paper illustrates how qualitative research can illuminate and generate understanding in a specific context. In many cases, the ideas and concepts that arise from qualitative research will be transferable to other contexts.

BOX 3.1: QUESTIONS TO ASK YOURSELF ABOUT A QUALITATIVE INTERVIEW STUDY

When reading a qualitative interview paper, always ask:

- Who undertook the interviews?
- Where were the interviews conducted?
- Who were the participants?
- How likely were the participants to be able to provide rich data for the study?
- How were the data analysed?
- Do the findings provide rich, contextual data?

REFLECTIONS FROM ONE OF THE PAPER'S AUTHORS

We were able to make contact with Gunilla Borglin, the lead author of this paper. Gunilla provided very generous feedback on a draft of this chapter, which we have summarised here:

It is a very relevant reflection that in this study we had no control of the managers for the 37 care centres for older people that we approached, or of what difference it would have made to our results if we had been able to recruit informants from a majority of them instead of from 10 centres out of 37. What we know is that 10 managers decided to forward our information letter to their RNs. Hence, all their RNs got the study information and decided by themselves that they wished to contact us or not (without their manager knowing if they did or did not). Ten RNs contacted us after having read the information letter and expressed their

(Continued)

interest to participate. Information was not given about which care centre these informants worked at as there would have been a high likelihood that informants could have been identified, as there were only one or two RNs at each care centre.

We agree that the terms used can be confusing – 'themes' and 'sub-themes' should have been replaced with 'categories' and 'sub-categories', and both a latent and manifest content analysis took place. We used a descriptive qualitative design, as understood from Sandelowski, so content analysis and the term 'categories' do not exclude interpretation.

SUGGESTED READING

Polit, D. and Beck, C. (2021) *Essentials of Nursing Research*. Alphen aan den Rign: Wolters Kluwer.
Sandelowski, M. (2010) What's in a name? Qualitative description revisited. *Research in Nursing & Health*, 33(1): 77–84.

4 A grounded theory paper

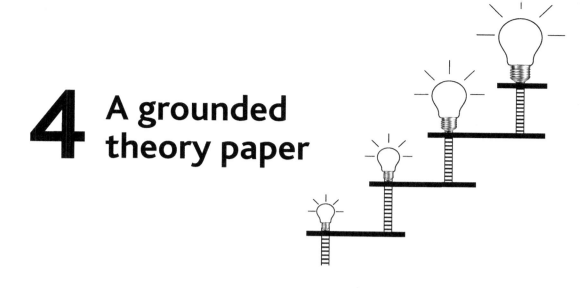

What is grounded theory?

Grounded theory is a specific method for doing qualitative research. It is undertaken when researchers want to understand the reasons and explanations for something; for example, a question suitable for a grounded theory study might be, 'Why do people manage their health concerns in a certain way?' To investigate this, researchers would collect rich in-depth data in order to develop a theory about how people manage their concerns, which can provide useful insights for those developing interventions to support them.

Grounded theory was one of the first qualitative methods to be specified. It was developed in the 1960s, an era dominated by the quantitative research approach. At this time, conducting research was largely synonymous with testing ideas through deductive quantitative methods. Grounded theory is widely accepted as the first documented and systematic approach to the collection and analysis of qualitative data. It was originally developed by Glaser and Strauss (1967) and first published in the classic text *The Discovery of Grounded Theory*; this work was the result of a research study exploring the experience of dying patients in a hospital setting. From this, the authors outlined a new method for examining qualitative phenomena in a systematic manner to generate understanding and theory. This qualitative method involves a structured approach to the sampling of participants, data collection and analysis. Glaser and Strauss (1967) therefore helped to enforce a recognisable process for a particular qualitative method which could help counter existing criticism about the unstructured (and, by implication, unreliable) nature of qualitative research. Since the work of Glaser and Strauss, other authors have offered alternative processes for doing grounded theory, for example Charmaz (2014).

In this chapter, we introduce you to a grounded theory study. We will discuss what grounded theory is, why researchers might choose to adopt a grounded theory method for their study and what this might mean for the conduct of the study and the results. The grounded theory paper we will explore in this chapter is:

> Mako, T., Svanäng, P. and Bjerså, K. (2016) Patients' perceptions of the meaning of good care in surgical care: A grounded theory study. *BMC Nursing*, 15(1): article no. 47.

This group of researchers were interested in developing a model, or theory, about the meaning of good surgical care, which could be used and applied within surgical nursing.

Get yourself a copy of the paper, read it through, then work/read through the rest of the chapter, finding the points we identify in the paper: https://link.springer.com/article/10.1186/s12912-016-0168-0

Scan the QR code to be taken straight to the paper.

What does the abstract and information about the authors tell me?

The abstract (and title) of the paper informs us that the paper is reporting a grounded theory study and that interviews were undertaken in order to collect data to address the study aim. The work of the research methodologist Charmaz is referred to, indicating the specific approach to grounded theory that was used in this study. We will discuss this in more detail throughout this chapter. The abstract also provides a summary of the results and conclusions in relation to the study aim.

ABSTRACT

Background

Patients in surgical care have reported a fear of being discharged prior to sufficient recovery and a lack of control of their situation. Establishing the patient–nurse relationship is essential in the context of the care. The Swedish National Board of Health and Welfare has established indicators for good care for comparison, evaluation and improvement of the quality of the health care system. These indicators are knowledge-based, appropriate, safe, effective and equal health care, as well as care within a reasonable time and patient-centred care. Current core competences in nursing education include quality improvement, patient-centred care, teamwork and collaboration, using evidence-based practice, safety and informatics. This study investigates patients' perceptions of the meaning of good care in inpatient surgical care.

Methods

Grounded theory according to Charmaz was chosen as the study design. Interviews were conducted with 13 patients from six surgical wards in the south of Sweden in 2014–2015.

Results

The results showed that patients in surgical care perceived good care as being safe, as they were vulnerable and anxious. This could be achieved through accessible care, reliable care, caring attitudes and participating in one's own care. Patient participation was achieved by information and education and the possibility to affect their care.

Conclusion

Patients need safety to experience good care. Caring attitudes and patient participation can be attained through patient-centred care. Bedside handover can improve patients' perceptions of accessible care and reliable care and can increase patient participation. Continuously maintaining competence and using evidence-based practice are needed to achieve reliable care.

Keywords: Evidence-based practice, Good care, Nurse, Patient participation, Patient-centred care, Quality improvement, Surgical care

The paper's authors are nurse academics at the University of Lincopling and Gotenburg in Sweden. We are told that one of the authors undertook the study as part of a master's-level degree. We could assume that the additional authors are part of the master's student's supervisory team.

Is there a clear research question or aim addressed by the research?

In this paper, the title is written as a statement indicating the study topic: *Patients' perceptions of the meaning of good care in surgical care*. In addition to the title, you should expect to find a research question or aim of the study stated in the main text. Sometimes the aim or research question is stated at the end of the introduction or background section. In this paper, it is at the start of the methods section.

METHODS

Aim

The aim of this study was to investigate patients' perceptions of the meaning of good care in inpatient surgical care.

In the introduction, the authors explain the full rationale for the study. They discuss what is currently understood about the concept of good care and they highlight a gap in the evidence: that the concept had not been fully explored within a surgical context and hence the need for their study.

How was the study designed?

This is a grounded theory study, following the particular approach taken to grounded theory by Charmaz (2014). Charmaz's work (2014) is an adaptation of the work of Glaser and Strauss (1967) and is a well-used and accessible method of doing grounded theory which has been published as a textbook outlining the practical steps required.

DESIGN

Grounded theory was chosen as the methodological approach and design based on the assumptions and interpretations presented by Charmaz [16].

The aim of grounded theory is, as its name suggests, to generate theory. Grounded theorists are not just interested in the description of a phenomenon but also aim to produce a theory from the qualitative data and subsequent analysis; the end result is theory generation. The data is collected from participants who are selected for their relevance to the aim or research question: a concept known as theoretical sampling. Data is collected until no new findings are emerging that might inform the theory: a concept known as theoretical saturation. Data is analysed by a process called constant comparison analysis: an inductive approach whereby data from different interviews are repeatedly compared with each other for the identification and development of categories, which then inform the development of a theory explaining the phenomenon or problem in the research question. This is an important concept to remember when you are reading a grounded theory study: the paper should result in the development of theory rather than concluding with a rich description of the phenomenon.

Charmaz (2014) has taken the principles of Glaser and Strauss's (1967) work and developed an approach in which the philosophy and methods differ from the original methods. For example, in Glaser and Strauss's original method, researchers were advised not to undertake a literature review prior to undertaking the study – contrary to what is required prior to most other study designs and research approaches. Their rationale for this was to prevent prior knowledge from influencing the data analysis or interpretation. However, Charmaz does not take this approach.

Mako et al.'s (2016) study was designed according to the principles of grounded theory (using Charmaz's approach) as the research team was interested in finding out about what good care meant to patients in surgical care. That is, they were interested not only in developing an understanding of how patients perceived good care, but also in developing a theory of how good care is established. Grounded theory was therefore an appropriate qualitative approach as they wanted to develop a theory. In order to do this, the three essential concepts of grounded theory – theoretical sampling, theoretical saturation and constant comparison analysis (see Table 4.1) – were present in the study.

BOX 4.1: GROUNDED THEORY STUDY

In a grounded theory study, you would expect to see the three concepts of: theoretical sampling, theoretical saturation and constant comparison analysis. However, these concepts are not only used within grounded theory. In particular, the concepts of saturation and constant comparison analysis are common to many qualitative research studies. Constant comparison analysis is a popular method of data analysis and is used independently from a grounded theory study.

Mako et al. (2016) identified potential participants through theoretical sampling. This means that, rather than identifying all the participants prior to the start of the study and planning ahead when to conduct the interviews, participants (of particular types) were recruited throughout the study, in order to meet the study's needs. The recruitment plan was not pre-determined. Interested participants were included in the data collection if they had experiences or characteristics that might help fill the gaps that emerged from the researchers' initial understanding of the data collected. This is a particular way of sampling and cannot be pre-determined as it depends on the emerging findings. It is generally unique to grounded theory.

In this study, data were collected via in-depth interviews with participants. Interviews are a common approach to data collection in qualitative research and can be undertaken face to face (in person), via telephone or virtually. Within grounded theory, however, researchers consider field notes and memos made during and after the interviews as data as well, and so they also look at these during data analysis along with what was said.

Linked to the concept of theoretical sampling is the concept of theoretical saturation, in which data collection ceases when saturation is reached: in other words, when new interviews do not reveal any new data or ideas relating to the topic of interest – the developing theory. Mako et al. (2016) report that five participants were excluded due to data saturation; that is, these individuals met the study's inclusion criteria, but it was not felt that any new data would arise from these five additional interviews.

> The gathering of data continued as long as there was no saturation. No new dimensions or properties emerged in the categories in the analysis of the tenth interview. Three more interviews were held in which no further or deeper data were obtained but only confirmations of previous findings. This was interpreted as saturation.

Finally, data was analysed using constant comparison analysis, a process of analysis in which data collected in the interviews is compared and contrasted with data from the other interviews in order to develop understanding of the data, which then leads to the identification of categories and the generation of theory.

What questions might be asked in a grounded theory study?

If a qualitative research study is aligned to a particular method – in this case, grounded theory – you would expect the questions asked during data collection to reflect this. In previous chapters, we have discussed how the questions in a qualitative study are designed to generate a rich and in-depth discussion. In a grounded theory study, questions should facilitate the generation of theory. In this study, the researchers were interested in finding out what good surgical care consists of, and questions asked of participants were designed to illicit data about this. Mako et al. (2016) describe how the interview questions were initially semi-structured and open-ended but were later adjusted to meet the needs of the study. This allowed the interviewer to explore areas according to the theoretical direction of the emerging data, and the evident gaps, in order to achieve the study aims. They report that the questions were not altered after the tenth interview. This is in line with the grounded theory method.

> As the interviews continued, the interview guide was adapted by adjusting the questions to follow the theoretical direction and to fill the gaps in the data to reach the study aim [16].

Is the interview schedule or topic guide made available to the reader?

As discussed in Chapter 3, the interview schedule in a qualitative interview is not intended to be a script to be adhered to but a guide to prompt exploratory questions. Mako et al. (2016) report two topic areas that were asked in every interview: whether the patient could describe a situation in which they experienced good care and a situation in which they experienced poor care. These questions were key to enabling the participants to describe both positive and negative experiences and would have been the trigger for further questions:

- Can you describe a situation during your stay where you experienced good care?
- Can you describe a situation during your stay where you experienced poor care?

It is important to note that, although safety is a clear outcome of this study, the researchers did not specifically ask about this aspect of care. Safety issues were identified by participants as an attribute of good and bad care, which enabled the researchers to develop the concept of safety within their findings.

Who was invited to participate in the study?

In Chapter 3, we discussed how sample sizes in qualitative research tend to be smaller than in quantitative studies because the aim is not to generalise from the findings but to generate insight and to report on the range of experiences. In this study, the overall aim was to generate theory. It almost goes without saying that those invited to a study need to meet the needs of the study. In this case, participants needed to meet the criterion of having had recent experience of surgical nursing care in one of two hospitals in Sweden. The inclusion criteria for participants can be found in the section on 'Setting and Participants':

Inclusion criteria were patients cared for in a surgical ward between a minimum of 3 days and a maximum of 30 days, being discharged from the ward less than 2 months previously, being able to speak and understand Swedish, and provision of verbal and written consent. Exclusion criteria were transfer to and discharge from another hospital or clinic, and cognitive impairment.

Potential participants needed to have been an inpatient for between three and 30 days. Recent care was defined as occurring within the previous two months: this time limit was in place so that participants were able to readily recall the care discussed in order to prevent 'recall bias'. It is important to note that most qualitative research relies on the memory of those participating; it is also well known that memory is not infallible (Blakey et al., 2019) and this needs to be considered in the analysis.

We can see in Mako et al.'s study that the participants comprised 13 people who had recently experienced surgical nursing care in Sweden, although they do not mention which type of surgery. In this grounded theory study, applying the concept of saturation meant that after interviewing 13 people, no new data relating to the topic was emerging from the interviews. Saturation, when appropriately applied, can create the reassurance that the sample size was large enough to answer the research question. The extent to which the generated theory can be applied in other countries will be discussed later in this chapter.

Who undertook the interviews?

In any study using interview methods, attention should be given to who undertook the interviews and where these took place. This is particularly so in qualitative studies where skill is required to carry out qualitative interviewing, due to their less structured nature. The quality of data generated by the interviews is, to some extent, dependent on the skills of the interviewer. In Mako et al.'s (2016) study, all the researchers are experienced surgical nurses, indicating that they had a good understanding of the research topic; however, it could be argued that they may have had a pre-existing view on what good surgical nursing care looked like and may have looked for this in the data. This is discussed in the paper and strategies were in place to reduce any subsequent risk of bias – for example, any preconceptions or prejudices held by the researchers that might affect data collection and analysis were discussed before data collection started, as well as during analysis. Further, information about their prior experience in interviewing is not provided.

Finding the right interviewer can be a difficult balance. If an interviewer is fully immersed in the area of study, they may inadvertently lead an interview in a certain direction; equally, a researcher who has no experience in an area might miss cues in the conversation that could provide a useful lead into further data. We are told that two researchers participated in the initial three interviews in order to provide each other with feedback. It is reasonable to assume that one of these researchers was the candidate for the educational award. None of the researchers appeared to have any connection with either of the hospitals where the study took place.

How did they analyse the results?

The purpose of data analysis in a qualitative study is to make sense of a large amount of (usually) narrative data: despite using small sample sizes, the volume of data generated can be large in qualitative studies. The analysis of data in a grounded theory study follows a well-defined process which is well described in this paper. Rather than waiting until all of the interviews are completed, data analysis commences once some initial interviews have been undertaken. This allows the process of theoretical sampling to take place along with checking for theoretical saturation. Interviews are transcribed, read and initial codes applied to the data (to 'label' it) before subsequent interviews take place. This allows researchers to reflect on the emerging data and consider whether additional questions need to be asked in subsequent interviews in order to shed more light on the research question, or whether particular types of respondents need to be interviewed. Mako et al. (2016) transcribed all the interviews word for word, including pauses and laughter. This level of detail is not always included in transcripts but was used here in order to achieve an understanding of context. Tentative initial coding was conducted before more focused coding to identify a theoretical direction. Focused coding was completed after each interview and then compared with previous initial codes and focused codes.

The process of constant comparison (the method of data analysis used in grounded theory studies) involves the comparison of data across all of the interviews in order to develop categories. Constant comparison continues until all of the interviews have been conducted and analysed. If an initial code has been applied to a section of data, this data is compared to other data where the same or similar code has been applied. This can lead to the revision of a code if, on reflection, the code does not fit the data very well: so that piece of data might be removed from that code and given a new label. This continual comparison across data or interviews is undertaken to create new categories or to fit data into existing categories. As such, Lincoln and Guba (1985: 342) describe a dynamic back and forth between the data in different interviews which gives the 'analyst confidence that he or she is converging on some stable or meaningful data set'.

The process of constant comparison analysis is firmly rooted in grounded theory. However, it is a process that is widely used in studies using other qualitative approaches, so do not be surprised if you find this concept applied in studies that are not aligned to a grounded theory method. There are also other approaches to data analysis in qualitative research such as thematic analysis (Braun and Clark, 2006), which we discuss in the next chapter. Constant comparison analysis has been rigorously applied by Mako et al. (2016). They give a detailed account of their analysis in the section titled 'Data analysis and saturation'.

DATA ANALYSIS AND SATURATION

The researchers transcribed all the records verbatim, unidentified and numbered. Rules for transcription were set prior to data collection. Laughs and pauses were noted in the transcriptions. The analysis was made according to Charmaz [16]. The analysis starts with an initial coding, which means separating segments of the data and labeling them with simple and precise words. These codes are tentative and the researchers should maintain an open mind during the analysis, stay close to the data while coding and constantly compare data with data. The initial coding includes looking for implicit actions and meanings, crystallising the significance in the data and identifying gaps in the data. In focused coding, the initial codes are used to sort and analyse the data and to identify a theoretical direction. The codes that reveal patterns and best account for the data serve as focused codes. Here, focused coding was done after each interview and then compared with previous initial codes and focused codes. In the process of theory building, the focused codes were analysed and theoretical categories were created. These categories gave a theoretical direction to the interviews. An example of the analysis process is shown in Table 1 [Figure 4.1].

How did they present the results?

In qualitative research, the analysed data are usually presented in the form of a narrative which is typically supported by indicative quotes, ideally from a range of participants. We can look at the quotes to see if they reflect and represent the results of the analysis. As readers, we can also check that quotes have come from a range of participants by looking at the study identification numbers linked to each quote. If all the quotes came from just two or three participants, we might question the quality of the data from other participants – we might wonder whether the analysis was based on the views of all participants or just a select group. If no study identification numbers are given, then we cannot make this judgement. Mako et al. (2016) used quotes from a good range of participants.

In grounded theory, in addition to the narrative, the theoretical contribution should also be evident. Mako et al. (2016) describe the categories that emerged from the data. These are 'accessible care', 'reliable care', 'caring attributes, information and education', and 'possibility to affect the care'. Mako et al. (2016) synthesised these into a model of good surgical care (Figure 1 in the paper), in which good care encompasses accessible and reliable care, administered with a caring attitude through information and education to patients who can influence or participate in the care provided, and in doing so that care enables patients to feel safe. This model (which is not a fully developed theory) argues that patients feel safe when care is accessible, reliable and delivered by caring staff who facilitate patient participation in their own care.

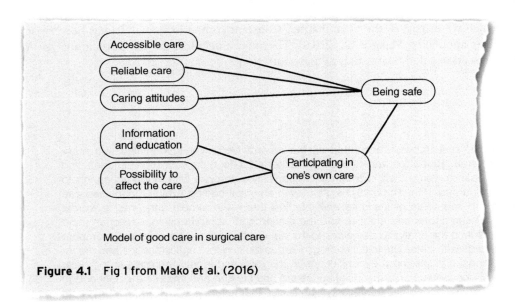

Model of good care in surgical care

Figure 4.1   Fig 1 from Mako et al. (2016)

Was the study ethical?

It is always important to consider the ethics of any study, even though, in the vast majority of cases, research proposals are put before an ethics committee for scrutiny prior to the study being undertaken. Despite this, additional scrutiny by the reader is important if only to reassure yourself that you understand the ethics of the paper you are reading.

The issue of ethical recruitment to research is always worthy of consideration. The Declaration of Helsinki (2013) emphasises that when seeking informed consent prior to research, researchers should be 'particularly cautious if the potential subject is in a dependent relationship with the physician or may consent under duress' (article 27).

In Chapter 3, we discussed the ethics of recruiting staff to participate in research and how they should feel no obligation to do so. In this study, we need to consider the recruitment of patients who are generally considered to be a more vulnerable group and might find it difficult to decline an invitation to participate. Mako et al. (2016) reassure us that potential participants had to opt into the study rather than opt out of it. In other words, those who were interested in participating were asked to contact the researchers; potential participants were not contacted directly by the researchers themselves. This is to ensure that those entering the study had a genuine interest in doing so and did not experience any coercion or pressure from either the clinical or research team to take part. We are told that 24 patients responded with an expression of interest in the study and that 13 patients eventually took part. Regarding other ethical aspects of the study, we are told that informed consent was obtained from all participants and that data was stored in accordance with data protection legislation.

How confident can we be of the results of the study?

In this study, the researchers aimed to develop a theory about the meaning of good care from the perspective of the patient. They achieved this through the grounded theory process, although they recognised the limitations in transferring their findings to other settings, and perhaps other countries. Findings from all research need to consider the context in which the study was undertaken as health care practices and systems differ both within and across countries and even within hospitals, depending on the ward culture. As described in the previous chapter, the confidence we have in a qualitative study comes from the transparency about each of its steps undertaken and from the explicit quality markers of the study, such as those identified by Lincoln and Guba (1985). Mako et al. (2016) followed a recognised method for doing a grounded theory study, as described by Charmaz (2014), and provided a clear account of the steps they undertook for the study. Readers of the study can identify the extent to which the findings can be transferred to a wider population of nurses and patients from other countries and settings.

In summary

In this chapter we have considered what you should be looking for when you read a grounded theory study. Grounded theory is a particular method for doing qualitative research. Researchers undertaking grounded theory use specific methodological concepts, including theoretical sampling, theoretical saturation and constant comparison analysis – you should look for these in the paper. For this study, the researchers followed the particular approach to grounded theory developed by Charmaz (2014). Grounded theory studies aim to generate or develop theory and we can see evidence of this in the model of safe surgical care advanced in this study, although it falls short of a full theory. The aim is not to generalise, in the way that we do from quantitative studies, but to seek an understanding. However, in many cases, the ideas and concepts that arise from qualitative research will be transferable to other contexts.

BOX 4.2: QUESTIONS TO ASK YOURSELF ABOUT A GROUNDED THEORY STUDY

When reading a grounded theory study, always ask:

- Who undertook the interviews?
- Where were the interviews conducted?
- Who were the participants?
- How likely were the participants to be able to provide rich data for the study? Was there evidence of theoretical sampling and theoretical saturation?
- How was the data analysed? Was constant comparison analysis used?
- Do the findings contribute to theory?

NOTE

We were unable to make contact with the authors of this paper.

SUGGESTED READING

Charmaz, K. (2015) Grounded theory. In J. A. Smith (ed.), *Qualitative Psychology: A Practical Guide to Research Methods* (3rd edition, pp. 81–110). London: Sage Publications.

5 A phenomenology paper

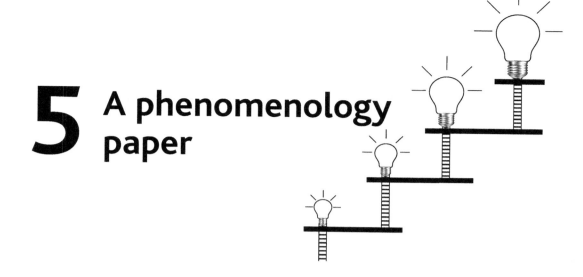

What is phenomenology?

> You never really understand a person until you consider things from his point of view, until you climb into his skin and walk around in it. (Harper Lee, *To Kill a Mockingbird*)

Phenomenology is another method that comes under the umbrella of qualitative research. It is based on the philosophical ideas of the importance of understanding lived experiences. It was developed in the early 1900s, for example by Husserl and Heidegger (Moustakas, 1994; Ranse et al., 2020), and has more recently been developed into a research method by many different researchers. Like grounded theory, phenomenology is a named method for a particular type of qualitative research – we use phenomenology when we are aiming to achieve an understanding of the direct experiences of those living with the phenomenon of interest. Phenomenology aims at describing the common meaning of lived experiences for several individuals, synthesising the experiences reported by individuals to a central meaning, or the 'essence' of the experience. This is important as we might assume that we understand what something is like from another person's perspective, whereas, in reality, our perspective might be very different. Understanding the perspectives and experiences of the patient or client, relative or health care professional is important in health care if services are to meet the needs of those who receive or deliver care. We will explore the philosophy of phenomenology further in this chapter.

The phenomenological paper we will explore in this chapter is:

Bragadottir, G. H., Halldorsdottir, B. S., Ingadottir, T. S. and Jonsdottir, H. (2018) Patients and families realising their future with chronic obstructive pulmonary disease: A qualitative study. *Journal of Clinical Nursing*, 27: 57–64.

What does the abstract and information about the authors tell me?

The abstract should be a concise account of the study that provides enough information to enable you to assess whether to access the paper in full. In the title, we are told that the study is qualitative, but the abstract is more specific, describing the study design as interpretive phenomenology. From this abstract, we know that the study aims to explore the experiences of patients and relatives living with, and learning about, having chronic obstructive pulmonary disease (COPD). The abstract tells us why the study has been done (the background), the method of data collection, who took part, and the headline findings, as well as a concise conclusion.

ABSTRACT

Aims and objectives

To gain insight into the lived experience of learning about having chronic obstructive pulmonary disease for patients and their families.

Background

Chronic obstructive pulmonary disease often progresses for years. Adjustment to declining health is gradual, and the disease may have developed considerably when health care is sought and people are diagnosed. Reaching patients at early stages is necessary to delay progression of the disease.

Design

Interpretive phenomenology.

Methods

Data were collected in four family focus group interviews ($N = 37$) and a sub-sample of eight family-dyad interviews. Patients were eight men, and 14 women aged 51–68 years. Majority of the patients ($n = 19$) were at GOLD grades II and III, with three at grade IV. The family members were eight men, and seven women aged 29–73 years. Data were collected between June–November 2012.

Results

Five, not mutually exclusive themes, revealed a long and arduous process of learning about and becoming diagnosed with chronic obstructive pulmonary disease and how unaware participants were of the imminent threat that the disease imposes on life. The themes were as follows: burden of shame and self-blame, enclosed in addiction, living in parallel worlds, realising the existence of the disease and a cry for empathy.

Conclusions

Learning about and realising the existence of chronic obstructive pulmonary disease and what it entails at the present time and in the future was bleak for the participants. The patients tended to put aside the thought of being a person with chronic obstructive pulmonary disease and defer actions that might halter progression of the disease, particularly to quit smoking.

The authors are from the University of Iceland and the University Hospital of Iceland. Two of the authors are clinical nurse specialists working in the area of respiratory disease. Another author is the head of the academic department section for chronically ill adults. Later in the paper, we learn that the first author was a master's student at the time of the study.

Is there a clear research question or aim addressed by the research?

The aim of the study is clearly stated in its own titled section:

2.1 AIM OF THE STUDY

To explore patients' and their families' lived experience of learning about having COPD.

Later in the paper, in the methods section, the authors provide a research question: '*What is the experience of learning about having COPD for patients and families?*' It is important to note that the authors are not directly interested in the patients' experience of the disease – as might be expected at first glance – but about how patients and their families learned about the disease, although the two concepts are connected and can be difficult to separate from each other.

The title of the paper, 'Patients and families realising their future with chronic obstructive pulmonary disease', reflects the findings, rather than the aim, of the research; remember that the stated aim was to gain insight into patients' and relatives' experiences of learning about having COPD. This is a good example of why it is important, when searching for papers on a given topic, not to restrict your search to key terms arising in the title of the paper only, as the title may relate to a key finding rather than the aim of the paper. Creative titles can be eye-catching when you are scanning down a contents list of a journal, but can make the paper less accessible if you are running a formal literature search focused only on titles.

How was the study designed?

This study aligns itself to the philosophy of phenomenology, describing itself as an interpretive phenomenological study. The term phenomenology refers to the school of philosophical inquiry, originating in the early 1900s from the work of Edmund Husserl (1859–1938) and further developed in the work of Heidegger (1889–1976) to explore the meaning of being. Both philosophers emphasised the importance of studying things as they appear, rather than of making assumptions. Thus, the aim of phenomenology is to put already held subjective ideas about phenomena on hold, whilst more objective observations about the nature of the phenomena are developed. Phenomenology is a critical approach that requires the researcher to revisit their understanding of a phenomenon and to explore the possibility of new meaning, or to authenticate previous meaning. As such, phenomenology is often regarded as a philosophy rather than an actual research method.

There are different approaches to phenomenology. For example, Husserl held the belief that phenomena should be looked at with no preconceived ideas so that any such preconceived ideas are bracketed (or separated) from the current knowledge of the observer, whereas Heidegger did not believe in the idea of bracketing. You might recall from the previous chapter that similar discussions are had regarding awareness of the background literature in grounded theory. Other philosophers continued the debate. For example, Merleau Ponty reignited the concept of bracketing, whereas Gadamer followed more closely the work of Heidegger and emphasised the importance of interpretation rather than a fundamental focus on description. From these examples, we can see that phenomenology is not one clear approach but a combination of a variety of approaches that have developed over the years. A good description of the work of these philosophers is provided by Ranse et al. (2020).

It is therefore not surprising, given these differing views among philosophers, that there are several methods for doing research that have developed from these philosophies of phenomenology. Research methodologists who have applied the philosophical principles of phenomenology to their work include Colaizzi (1978), Giorgi (1985), Benner (1994b) and Van Manen (2017). They have attempted to clarify a research method that stayed true to the principles of their understanding of phenomenology, and have seminal texts that guide researchers through a method for undertaking research that is reflective of a phenomenological position. However, each has a slightly different emphasis and interpretation – for example, Colaizzi and Giorgi focus on a descriptive phenomenology (Colaizzi, 1978; Giorgi, 1985), whilst Van Manen and Benner advocate an interpretative approach (Benner, 1994b; Van Manen, 2017). None are right or wrong, and you will often find these research-ers referred to in nursing research that follows a phenomenological approach. It is beyond the scope of this chapter to discuss these philosophers and researchers further, but this will alert you to the complexities in the development and use of phe-nomenology in nursing research, and the various approaches and discussion that you might encounter regarding ways of doing phenomenology – so don't be surprised if things look slightly different in another phenomenology paper.

Bragadottir et al. (2018) refer to the work of Benner (1994a) and Leonard (1994) to justify the approach they adopted for their study but, as is often the case in a jour-nal article, do not offer a detailed account of why they chose this particular method and the implications of this for their study or findings. They also refer to the work of Merleau-Ponty without giving a clear rationale for the reference. We are told that the study is an interpretative phenomenology; that is, the researchers are attempting to interpret the experiences rather than simply describe them.

3.1 DESIGN

Premises of interpretive phenomenology were used to elicit the meaning of learning about having COPD for individuals and their families (Benner, 1994; Leonard, 1994). Attention is directed towards what it means to be a person with an emerging lung disease with all-embracing nicotine addiction and breathing difficulties that interact with personal concerns, habits, relationships and culture. The notion of embodiment further underscores the uniqueness of the human body, through which the person lives, experiences and interacts with the world (Merleau-Ponty, 1945/2012).

Phenomenology has been a popular approach in nursing research due to its empha-sis on understanding phenomena, and the experiences of patients and families, so that we can develop care that better reflects or meets their needs. Yet, it has been subject to much debate, for example in the work of Crotty (1996), who, on review-ing a selection of nursing research papers, argued that much nursing research has deviated from the original intention of phenomenology, which was to seek the essence and understanding of the phenomenon under investigation. Instead, this 'new' phenomenology focuses on the researcher researching the experiences of oth-ers (for example, patients or health care professionals) rather than the researcher's own experiences (Barkway, 2001), and hence has diverged from the original intent of phenomenology. Bragadottir et al. (2018) designed a phenomenological study to explore the experiences of patients and their relatives of learning about having COPD. This study therefore reflects the 'new' phenomenology, where the phenomenon is explored through the standpoint of those interviewed.

The experiences of patients and their relatives of living with COPD were collected through discussion in family focus groups and family-dyad interviews rather than through individual interviews. Data was collected from participants who were already participating in another ongoing research study. The sample is a sub-sample of those taking part in a randomised controlled trial – which is interesting, but not uncommon – so we need to consider how representative the participants are of the wider population of people with COPD. It is also important to consider the impact of this on the overall findings.

There were four focus group interviews: two with participants from the experimental group and two from the control group. Seven to 10 people participated in each focus group. Eight family-dyad interviews were conducted: two where the patient was male and six where the patient was a woman.

The rationale for group interviews is not given in the paper but we might assume that group discussion was selected to generate a discussion, reflective of shared experiences. Focus groups are a method of data collection often used in qualitative studies. The aim of a focus group is that the discussion itself generates reflection on the part of the participants which triggers new ideas in other participants which might not arise in a one-to-one interview; it is the interactions in the focus group that are of interest, rather than the individual statements of the participants. Hence, focus groups are often used when researchers anticipate that discussion will add depth to the data collected. A counter-argument would be that the experience of learning about having COPD is deeply personal and may not be amenable to group discussion.

What questions might be asked in a phenomenological study?

The questions asked of participants in a phenomenological study are generally open questions that are aimed to facilitate the participants' description of their experiences. Bragadottir et al. (2018) inform us that they sought to obtain depth when eliciting meaning of the experiences through the questions posed, and that they aimed to generate conversation about the experiences and the meaning in day-to-day life when living with COPD. Given the findings of the focus groups, the researchers were interested in further exploring the concept of shame, and so this was followed up in the family-dyad interviews.

Is the interview schedule or topic guide made available to the reader?

The focus group guide is helpfully available to the reader in Table 2 of the paper. You will see that most of the questions are open questions which would encourage discussion; however, one of the questions asks whether the participant had experienced shame or guilt because of their lung disease. This is a direct, closed question which might just generate a 'yes' or 'no' answer. With a topic guide such as this, the researcher does not have to ask the questions exactly as written but needs to ensure that they cover the topics listed during the focus group or interview. What is not clear from the paper is whether this same guide was used within the family-dyad interviews as well.

TABLE 2 Family-dyad focus group interview guide

1. What is of most importance to you regarding the lung disease; what are your main concerns?

2. How do the influences of the lung disease manifest in your daily life?

3. What feelings surface when you think about the lung disease?

4. How did you get to know about the existence of the lung disease; what kind of indications were there and what were the influences?

5. Have you experienced shame or guilt because of the lung disease?

6. How does the family talk about the lung disease?

7. What do you do/say to people when you cannot do something because of the lung disease or otherwise you would like to tell people about the disease?

8. What kind of health care do you consider of importance to people with beginning COPD?

Figure 5.1 Table 2 from Bragadottir et al. (2018)

Who was invited to participate in the study?

Participants were invited from a group of people who had taken part in a randomised controlled trial (RCT), a study which investigated self-management treatment for COPD: that is, they had all taken part in research, having been previously identified as living with the disease and were subsequently invited to take part in an additional phenomenological study. We are told that participants were invited from both the control and experimental groups of the RCT. Although patients are allocated at random into either arm of the trial and we would expect the experiences of those in each arm to be similar up to the point of taking part in the RCT, the intervention arm in this trial was a self-management programme and hence might affect the experiences of the participants in this arm. We might also want to consider whether the views of those who took part in the RCT (regardless of which arm of the trial they were in) might have differed in some way to those who did not, and whether this might impact on the findings.

3.2 PARTICIPANTS AND SETTING

The participants were individuals with COPD and family members who had participated in a 1-year randomised controlled trial of a partnership-based self-management treatment (Jonsdottir et al., 2015). All patients in that study, who were accompanied by a family member (n = 30), were invited into this study.

Who undertook the interviews?

We have discussed in previous chapters how attention should be given to who undertook the interviews in a qualitative study. In this study, the interviews were carried out by the researchers who are clinicians and researchers in the clinical field. Based on this, we can assume that the interviewers were knowledgeable in the topic and could follow up with appropriate questioning in an interview situation. However, we should also consider whether they might have predisposing views of the phenomenon under study and ask how these were managed.

How did they analyse the results?

The data from the focus groups and family-dyad interviews was transcribed verbatim and analysed thematically. Thematic analysis, based on the work of Braun and Clark (2006), is a form of data analysis often used in qualitative research. The approach has similarities with constant comparison analysis discussed in the previous chapter, although there are differences. In a thematic analysis, researchers develop themes rather than categories, though these are developed in a similar way, by comparing and contrasting the qualitative data in a study.

Bragadottir et al. (2018) involved all the researchers in the initial analysis and identification of themes, which suggests increased rigour within the study as the analysis is undertaken by more than one person. The initial analysis of the data in this study was undertaken in the language of origin – Icelandic – after which the data was translated into English for the final analysis and preparation for publication. Perhaps a limitation might be translating the interviews before analysis, as sometimes nuances of the meaning of the language or conversation might have been lost.

All interviews were conducted in Iceland and transcribed verbatim. The first author undertook the analysis of the data with all authors actively contributing in conversations about a coherent presentation of the participants' experience (Benner, 1994). All authors discussed the themes to invite alternate interpretations and ensure logical flow of the findings, and principally to discuss the meaning of the data (Cutcliffe and McKenna, 1999; Kvale and Brinkmann, 2009).

As interpretation and analysis of data took place concurrently, the data analysis started in the first focus group interview. Along with the transcribed interviews, observation notes and authors' diaries were treated as text analogues (Benner, 1994; Kvale and Brinkmann, 2009). Preliminary data analysis was conducted in Iceland. Then the text was turned into English by the research team for final analysis of results with the help of an English translator. Engaging in the hermeneutic circle of understanding, interpretation and a thematic analysis were undertaken where commonalities and differences were revealed, and issues and patterns were analysed (Benner, 1994).

How did they present the results?

The purpose of a thematic analysis is to generate themes inductively from the data. That means that the researchers are not looking at the interview transcripts expecting to find certain things, rather they read the transcripts with an open mind and code sections of the text that they identify as relevant to the research question. These codes are then developed into themes.

Bragadottir et al. (2018) presents the results as five themes, and each is given a label or title. Sometimes titles for themes are self-explanatory or developed directly from quotations within the data. At other times, the titles might seem less immediately linked to the data. In this study, the theme titles are quite abstract: the researchers do not always explain the theme titles in detail and the included quotes don't always reflect the title either. The themes are presented in the paper as: the burden of shame, enclosed in addiction, living in a parallel world, cry for empathy, and the reality of the existence of the disease. Explaining theme titles can be very helpful to the reader. However, the authors do provide a narrative for the themes and support the themes with accompanying quotations:

4.3 LIVING IN PARALLEL WORLDS

The lung disease went more or less unrecognised in the daily life of the families. The family members were not aware of the many levels on which the disease afflicted the patients, and the patients kept their difficulties to themselves: 'I have this problem and I have to live with it.' Therefore, the patients tended to hide the disease both from themselves and others, even their closest family members.

We noted in the earlier chapters on papers reporting qualitative studies that supporting quotes should come from a range of the study participants rather than just one or two, and so it is helpful if an identifier (an identity number or a pseudonym) is attached to each quote to help us assess this. Identifiers were not included in Bragadottir et al. (2018) and so it is hard for us to judge whether or not these quotes came from a range of participants across the sample to inform the developing themes.

Was the study ethical?

This study included patients who were already recruited into another study: a randomised controlled trial. Given the importance of voluntary participation in research, we need to consider whether the participants felt any obligation to participate in the phenomenological study, having already been recruited into the RCT and being known to the researchers.

Another factor to consider is the potential risk of harm to participants. There are two possible aspects to this. First, participation in a study in which the possible suggestion that their lifestyle choices might have influenced their disease, could be an uncomfortable experience. Furthermore, the data was collected in focus groups or family-dyad interviews, with any self-disclosure being made to a group, including family members (as opposed to just to a single non-related interviewer). This is especially relevant considering that the researchers became particularly interested during the study in the concept of shame and guilt and how lifestyle choices might have contributed to the illness.

One of the fundamental principles that guides research ethics is informed consent. The consent to participate in a study implies that the participant accepts the potential for harm. We are not told whether the participants were warned that they would be specifically asked about the concepts of shame and guilt within a group context when they gave their consent to participate. However, we can be confident that the study had full ethical approval. Furthermore, it is important that everyone taking part in a study is assured that they cannot be identified once the study is written up.

3.4 ETHICAL CONSIDERATIONS

The Icelandic Data Protection Authority (2009020191BRA, 2009020191AT), The National Bioethics Committee (VSNb2009020016/03.15), the Primary Health Care of the Capital Area of Reykjavik (1A3g/23/845.1/LÓ/ló) and the manager of the pulmonary physicians' clinic granted permission for the study.

How confident can we be of the results of the study?

Through this phenomenological study, the researchers aimed to understand the experience of patients and families when they learn to live with a lung disease. Understanding this experience should help us to ensure that care delivery meets the related patient and family need. The researchers clearly describe the processes they undertook to ensure the rigour of the study, such as two researchers undertaking the data collection and the involvement of all of the authors in the data analysis. A total of four focus groups and eight family-dyad interviews were undertaken, which is likely to have provided adequate data for the analysis (although it is important to consider the type of information participants would be prepared to share in these contexts). The authors emphasised the need for honesty, accuracy and self-assertiveness, not only in undertaking the interviews but also in the data analysis. The results should provide an authentic picture of how participants learned to live with this lung disease, and the extent to which the findings can be transferred to a wider population of patients can be considered by the reader.

In summary

In this chapter we have summarised some of the key points you should consider when reading a paper about a phenomenological study. Phenomenological studies are designed to elicit the lived experiences from participants to enable a better understanding of what it is like to live with a certain condition, or in particular circumstances. The method needs to elicit detailed description of the lived experience and to analyse the data and present the findings in a way that is true to this experience. This type of approach is sometimes considered central to our understanding of the world of patients and therefore important to the work of nurses and other health care professionals.

BOX 5.1: QUESTIONS TO ASK YOURSELF ABOUT A PHENOMENOLOGICAL STUDY

When reading a phenomenological paper, always ask:

- Did the researchers follow a specific approach to phenomenology?
- Does the study focus on meaning?
- Who were the participants?
- How likely were the participants to be able to provide rich data for the study?
- Who undertook the interviews?
- Where were the interviews conducted?
- How were the data analysed?

REFLECTIONS FROM ONE OF THE PAPER'S AUTHORS

We were able to make contact with Helga Jonsdottir, the lead author of this paper. Helga provided very generous feedback on a draft of this chapter, which we have summarised here:

(Continued)

Thank you very much for using our paper in your book. I am very pleased with how you do this. I like how you address the shortcomings. There is a reference to Braun and Clarke about thematic analysis, but I do not find it illustrates well how we did the data analysis. We followed the work of Benner and refer to a chapter in her 1994 book – this was an essential part of our understanding and use of interpretative phenomenology in this study.

SUGGESTED READING

Krueger, R. A. and Casey, M. A. (2014) *Focus Groups: A Practical Guide for Applied Research* (5th edition). London: Sage Publications.

Ranse, T., Arbon, P., Cusack, L., Shabon, R. and Nicolls, D. (2020) Obtaining individual narratives and moving to an inter-subjective lived experience description: A way of doing phenomenology. *Qualitative Research*, 20(6): 945–959.

6 A randomised controlled trial paper

What is a randomised controlled trial?

A randomised controlled trial (RCT) is an experiment. It is a particular type of study undertaken when we want to find out if something works or not: whether it is effective. This might be a drug, a procedure or another type of intervention. In its most simple form, researchers administer the drug, procedure or other intervention to people who have been randomly assigned to one of two groups: an intervention group (who receive the intervention) or a control group (who receive standard care). Both groups are then followed up and any difference between the groups can feasibly be attributed to the drug, procedure or other intervention being tested. We can see that RCTs are very important in health care as it is vital that we know if our treatments and interventions are effective. In fact, criticism has been levelled at the absence of RCTs, and hence at an absence of evidence about the effectiveness, for well-accepted, commonly used treatments. For example, the evidence base for tonsillectomy is not as clear cut as we might think, despite it being a frequently carried out procedure (Windfurh, 2016).

A randomised controlled trial is a quantitative study, clearly fitting in the positivist paradigm where direct measurements and comparison take place (see Chapter 1 for a discussion of paradigms). The controlled manner in which the study is undertaken enables researchers to make direct comparisons between two or more similar groups of people who either receive the intervention or not. When seeking to find out whether an intervention works or not (or which intervention works best), we compare two (or more) existing interventions, or we compare a new intervention to either no intervention or a placebo intervention (a placebo is something that seems to be a 'real' medical treatment but is not). Comparison to usual care or 'treatment as usual' can be quite common in an RCT, especially when the intervention is more about an approach to treatment (such as a new service or a type of surgical procedure) rather than a drug. Ideally, the only difference between the groups is whether or not they receive the intervention of interest. In that way, any differences between the groups can be attributed to the intervention being tested. This makes it a rigorous study design and if we are looking to test the effectiveness of an intervention, we need to undertake an RCT. If we look for, but do not identify, any RCTs for a particular intervention, then we should conclude that the formal evidence base for it is likely to be weak; even an intervention that is long established and accepted as usual practice might not have an evidence base to underpin it. There are many different types of RCTs – the type used will depend on the nature of the question the researchers are trying to answer.

The randomised controlled trial we will explore in this chapter is:

Pulkkinen, M., Jousela, I., Engblom, J., Salantera, S. and Junttila, K. (2020) The effect of a new peri-operative practice model on length of hospital stay and on the surgical care process in patients undergoing hip and knee arthroplasty under spinal anaesthesia: A randomised clinical trial. *BMC Nursing*, 19: article no. 73.

Get yourself a copy of the paper, read it through, then work/ read through the rest of the chapter, finding the points we identify in the paper: https://bmcnurs.biomedcentral.com/ articles/10.1186/s12912-020-00465-3

Scan the QR code to be taken straight to the paper.

What does the abstract and information about the authors tell me?

The abstract should be a concise account of the study that provides enough information to help you decide if the paper might be useful for you and so whether to access it in full. From Pulkkinen et al.'s abstract, we know that the trial aims to explore the effect of a new peri-operative practice model on the length of stay and surgical care for patients undergoing arthroplastic hip or knee replacement surgery, compared to standard peri-operative care. So, participants were randomly allocated to either the new surgical model of practice or to standard peri-operative care: this sort of relation is sometimes described as comparison to 'usual care' or 'treatment as usual'. Patients' length of stay and other surgical outcomes were then monitored. The five authors are representative of different nursing and academic specialities which is indicative of a collaborative approach to the research.

Is there a clear research question or aim addressed by the research?

Although there is no specific research question, the title of the paper, 'The effect of a new peri-operative practice model on length of hospital stay and on the surgical care process in patients undergoing hip and knee arthroplasty under spinal anesthesia: A randomised clinical trial', reflects the aims of the trial which are stated as:

i. to explore the effect of a new peri-operative practice model (NPPM) on the length of stay and the time points of the surgical care process in patients undergoing total hip arthroplasty (THA) and total knee arthroplasty (TKA) under spinal anaesthesia, compared to those of patients in standard peri-operative care.

ii. to find out if there were different responses between the different subgroups.

Do note that in this study, RCT refers to 'randomised clinical trial' rather than 'randomised controlled trial'. As randomisation implies the allocation of participants to one group or another, and their comparison, the terms essentially mean the same thing.

In addition, the researchers provide a hypothesis at the end of the background section. A hypothesis is simply an idea, usually based on some evidence, that the researchers intend to test and can be used instead of a research question. In this paper, it was hypothesised that the intervention group would have a statistically significantly shorter mean length of stay than the control group. This hypothesis is then tested in the study. Do note, however, that only quantitative studies using direct and precise measurement can accurately test a hypothesis.

> In this study, we hypothesised that the intervention group would have statistically significantly shorter mean LOS than the control group. To our knowledge, there is limited research that examines how peri-operative, nurse-delivered interventions influence the LOS in patients undergoing THA and TKA.

The researchers had conducted a qualitative pilot study of the intervention previously with promising results relating to the patient experience, but wanted to explore its impact on length of stay and timings around the surgical process: that is, they sought quantifiable evidence to be able to justify the effectiveness of the intervention.

How was the study designed?

Most scientists consider that the only way we can truly find out if something works or not, or works better than current practice, is to do a randomised controlled trial.

There are lots of debates around the various aspects of trial design, such as who takes part in the trial (and therefore its representativeness and subsequent generalisability), or whether the setting up and running of the trial truly reflects the real world (hence questioning its applicability). However, the basic premise is well established: unless we do an RCT, we cannot know for sure whether an intervention or a treatment is effective. This is because randomisation reduces potential bias by seeking a balance in participant characteristics which could impact on differences in outcomes between the groups; this relates to both characteristics we know about and those we don't. This means that RCTs can provide a rigorous tool to examine cause–effect relationships between an intervention and an outcome. This is not possible with any other study design. This is why RCTs have become so important in health care – in fact, they are often called the 'gold standard' for those 'does it work?' questions and provide strong evidence for practice.

Pulkkinen et al. (2020) identified a 'does it work?' question: they wanted to find out if their new peri-operative practice model (NPPM) was effective at reducing length of stay and other factors associated with the quality of peri-operative care. This is an important question as length of stay is a critical factor for patients, staff and services, and a reduced length of stay has many benefits including reduced rates of infection and reduced costs associated with care. This helps illustrate why we should undertake trials of an intervention that might help to reduce overall time in hospital. We might feel intuitively that a particular approach to the delivery of care is a good thing; however, unless we test this out in a rigorous way, we will not know whether our intuitive ideas have led to the development of an intervention that is actually effective in practice.

Before conducting their RCT, the researchers carried out a qualitative pilot study involving 20 patients in order to assess patients' experience of the intervention they had developed. They did this in order to determine whether a study to test the effectiveness of the intervention was appropriate. This pilot identified that patients valued the intervention: they appreciated the one-to-one continuity of care from the assigned nurse and felt involved in their care. However, this was a pilot study only; the value of collecting only patients' experience data is limited in terms of assessing effectiveness. In order to determine whether an intervention is truly effective in reducing length of hospital stay, or other factors associated with quality of peri-operative care, a controlled experiment is required. As much as patients might appreciate and value continuity of care, the researchers wanted to know if the intervention had an effect on specific measurable outcomes such as length of hospital stay. Interestingly, outcomes such as decreased patient anxiety or increased knowledge were not measured in this trial, which you might find surprising for a nursing-led study.

The importance of the RCT can be seen here. We might think intuitively that it is a good idea to provide continuous nurse-led care throughout the whole peri-operative period, yet unless we formally test out this idea, using randomisation, we will not know for sure. Pulkkinen et al. (2020) were interested in knowing whether their intervention led to reduced length of stay and other surgical outcomes. That is, the researchers were not content with knowing the likely positive impact of the intervention on patient experience, or whether it is an intrinsic good in its own right;

they were interested in finding out whether it had an effect on specific measurable outcomes such as length of stay.

The design of a randomised controlled trial, in its basic form, is straightforward. You identify a group of people who are in the particular situation you want to study: in this case, patients who are about to undergo arthroplastic surgery. You divide them into two or more groups by a process of randomisation; randomisation means that participants have an equal chance of being allocated to either (or any) group. If there are two groups then one group receives the new intervention or treatment, and the other receives standard care or a placebo. There are other variations on this design. For example, where strict individual randomisation is not possible (i.e. randomisation of individual patients), a process called cluster randomisation can be used where randomisation occurs at a higher level such as the study site (e.g. ward, hospital or GP surgery). Where randomisation itself is not possible, a simple before and after design can be used to test an intervention, but this is a much weaker study design as, without the randomisation, it is not possible to determine what would have happened to the participants if they had not received the intervention. Studies which deviate from the controlled design of the RCT are often referred to as quasi-experiments and it is beyond the scope of this book to discuss all possible variations of design. Suggested further reading is indicated at the end of this chapter.

Pulkkinen et al. (2020) wrote, and made available, a protocol for their study. Research teams sometimes publish their trial protocols as journal papers or register them on nationally or internationally recognised databases (e.g. NIH at Clinical.Trials.gov, or ISRCTN at www.isrctn.com); Pulkkinen et al.'s (2020) protocol was registered on NIH at Clinical.Trials.gov and they provide us with the registration number (NCT02906033) so that we can access it. A protocol is the written, predefined method, or set of procedures, for the experiment: it is a bit like a recipe. It is a document that describes how a trial will be conducted (e.g. the objective, design, methodology, statistical considerations and trial organisation and management) and ensures the safety of the trial subjects and the integrity of the data collected.

Pulkkinen et al. (2020) wanted to test the NPPM intervention. The NPPM intervention was as follows: patients had a designated anesthesia nurse (AN) for their entire peri-operative period. This same designated nurse also visited the patient on the ward following their surgery. The focus of the NPPM was on the patients' personal and individual care needs, in order to enable emotional support, motivation to participate in self-care and continuity of care. Those in the control group received their usual care from the peri-operative nurses: this meant that they did not experience a level of continuity from the same nurse, nor did they receive a post-operative visit on the ward.

In an ideal world, the randomisation process should be undertaken using a computer-generated sequence where no one associated with the participant recruitment, data collection or analysis has any potential influence on the allocation of participants to either the intervention or control group. This ensures that it is down to complete chance whether a participant is allocated to the intervention or control group (or 'arm') of the trial. This is important as complete impartiality may be unrealistic by those running a trial who might, unconsciously or consciously, bias the allocation of participants into each arm of the trial, should they be given any role in this process.

In Pulkkinen et al. (2020), participants who were eligible to take part in the trial were invited to do so at their pre-operative outpatient appointment. They were randomised to receive either the NPPM intervention or their usual care. We are told that a randomisation sequence was performed by an independent third party and that those who had agreed to participate in the trial drew one of two cards which indicated which group they would be allocated to: the intervention group (NPPM) or the control group (usual care). From this, we assume that the cards were randomly ordered and, if they were placed in envelopes, that the envelopes were opaque so no one could see which group was on the card until the envelope was opened.

> Randomization was performed by an independent third party (a nurse at the outpatient clinic during the preoperative visit 2–3 weeks prior to scheduled operation). Eligible patients drew one of two cards; one indicated invitation to participate in the study and the other was blank indicating not participating in the study. Patients for the control group and the intervention group were by the group both recruited and scheduled for operation every other week. This stratification aimed to ensure that the patients in the two groups did not exchange information in the postoperative ward.

It is usual practice that the groups then received their allocated intervention and are then followed up to explore the pre-determined outcomes. Assuming the groups are big enough (group size is calculated through a process known as power calculation, discussed below), and that not too many people drop out of the trial part way through, any differences between the two groups can, in theory, be attributed to the new intervention or treatment, as all other differences between the groups are accounted for by randomising the participants and other factors associated with the trial design.

In an RCT, ideally neither the researchers nor the providers of the intervention know who is in which group, and the participants do not know which group they are in – this is usually called blinding. This can be difficult to achieve and is sometimes impossible – for example, depending on the type of intervention, it is almost impossible to blind those who provide the intervention, most often clinical staff. You can imagine that if the intervention was a drug, then it would be possible to blind those administering the drug or placebo, whereas if the intervention was a service, then it would not be possible to blind those providing the service. The reason why blinding is important is to manage the impact of any expectations associated with the treatment or intervention or control condition which could influence the outcome, over and above the impact of the intervention itself. For example, those allocated to the treatment or intervention group – if aware of this allocation – might 'expect' a particular reaction or response to the treatment or intervention. Likewise, those delivering the intervention or running the research might similarly be 'expecting' to see such reactions or responses and this could influence the process of data collection and/or data analysis. So, ideally, all are 'blind' to the group allocation of participants, but sometimes this can only be achieved for one or some of the parties involved.

Pulkkinen et al. (2020) describe their trial as 'single blind', implying that not all of the parties involved were blinded to participants' group allocation; elsewhere in the paper, they use different language meaning the same thing, referring to participants as being 'masked'. The intervention providers were not 'masked' or blinded, due to the nature of the intervention being tested. However, the researchers' process for actioning the randomisation ensured that participants in the intervention and control groups took part in the trial during alternate weeks so that the groups would not meet each other. Therefore, although those in the intervention group would be aware of the intervention and what it involved, those in the control group would not be aware of the exact type of care the intervention group received.

STUDY DESIGN

The study was a two-group parallel single-blind randomised clinical trial.

Once the participants are allocated to groups (ideally with neither the participant nor researcher knowing which group they are in), the intervention is delivered to the intervention group and withheld from the control group. Both groups are followed up, with those dropping out of the trial recorded alongside their reasons for dropping out: this is called attrition. For Pulkkinen et al. (2020), attrition was not a great concern as all follow-up data was collected from the participants' records, rather than directly from participants themselves, and this did not require any additional contribution from the participants. However, participants could still withdraw their consent for access to their records and patient deaths could occur before the end of the data collection period, meaning that complete datasets may not have been available for all participants.

What is assessed in a randomised controlled trial?

Once an RCT has been set up according to the principles outlined above, researchers follow up those in the intervention and control groups and monitor the outcomes of each group according to the trial protocol. Pulkkinen et al. (2020) wanted to establish whether those receiving the intervention experienced shorter lengths of time throughout the surgical care process, including: preparation time prior to surgery, surgery time, operating room time, recovery time and discharge from hospital. As mentioned earlier, the only primary outcome of interest was time; they did not collect data such as patient satisfaction or patient anxiety levels. Data was collected from the operating room management software and hospital information system for patients in both the intervention and control groups. In addition, demographic details were collected such as age, gender, procedure, day of operation and pre-operative general health status. This means that when participants agreed to take part in the trial, they agreed for the researchers to have access to their medical records in order to obtain data on their outcomes following surgery, regardless of whether they were randomised to the intervention or control group. In all RCTs, researchers need to decide what to measure, and what measurement tools to use in order to measure it, in order to assess which treatment is best. This might be a quality of life score, a pain score or even length of survival. Deciding on the outcome is a crucial step – the primary outcome should relate directly to the hypothesis, research question or aim. RCTs usually also collect data on additional outcomes of interest: these are called secondary outcomes.

In Pulkkinen et al.'s (2020) trial, they collected a lot of different measures but their primary outcome was length of stay (LOS) in days from hospital admission to hospital discharge. They were looking to see whether the intervention could make at least a half day's difference to the length of stay. We can deduce this from our reading of the paper because they used length of stay (LOS) to calculate how many potential participants they needed in the study, which we discuss below.

> The care process time points that were estimated were as follows: preparation time from the patient's arrival to the operating department to the administration of anesthesia agents (h), surgery time from incision to closing of the wound (h), operating room time from patient entrance to the operating room to patient exit from it (h), PACU time (h), recovery time from patient readiness for discharge from PACU to patient discharge from the hospital (h) and LOS from hospital admission to hospital discharge (days).

SAMPLE SIZE AND STATISTICAL METHODS

> The sample size requirement for comparing two LOS means was checked with power analysis (2-sided test) with $\alpha = 0.05$, $\beta = 0.9$, standard deviation $= 1.6$ and differences of means $= 0.5$ days. Sufficient sample size was determined to be $n = 217$ patients per group. For PACU time, it was determined as $n = 76$ patients per group (standard deviation $= 0.94$, differences of means $= 0.5$ h).

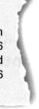

The number of participants that need to be recruited into a trial is determined by a statistical formula called a power calculation. This is based on the primary outcome for the study (the main factor or variable being measured). This is a crucial part of a trial's design, as if the trial is too small, any differences in outcome of the intervention may not be apparent and the study might inappropriately conclude that the intervention does not work, whereas, in fact, the numbers in the study were simply too small to demonstrate a clear finding. This is sometimes referred to as a type 1 error: where the null hypothesis (that is, the hypothesis that states that there is no difference in outcome for those who received the intervention and those who did not) is rejected prematurely due to inadequate numbers of people taking part. On the other hand, if the sample size is too large then questions arise around the ethics of continuing to randomise participants to receiving an intervention or not. Pulkkinen et al. (2020) used a power calculation in order to determine the number of participants needed in the study. They based this on the primary outcome measure, which was mean length of stay, and concluded that they would need 76 patients in each group.

Are the assessments made available to the reader?

It is standard practice for a list of the assessments or outcome measures used in a trial to be made available to the reader; sometimes the tools themselves are provided in an additional electronic file. The possibility of providing electronic files increases the transparency of data which would otherwise not be accessible to readers (unless the measures themselves have been published elsewhere). It may also be possible to look up the trial protocol to check on the outcomes (if the protocol has been published or registered). In Pulkkinen et al.'s (2020) trial, the assessments are reported in the text and listed in Table 2 of the paper.

Who was invited to participate in the study?

People attending a pre-operative outpatient appointment for elective total knee or total hip arthroplasty were invited to participate in the trial. These outpatient appointments took place 2–3 weeks prior to surgery, at which point potential participants would have given their informed consent to participate and to be randomised to either arm of the trial.

How did they analyse the results?

The purpose of the analysis of an RCT is usually to identify whether there are statistically significant differences in the outcomes between the different groups in the trial: the trial arms. The underlying principle is that if those undergoing hip or knee arthrosplasty who were randomly allocated to the two groups (the nurse-led intervention and the control group) were sufficiently similar at the start of the trial, any differences in the length of stay and other outcomes identified at the end could reasonably be attributed to the intervention: in this case, the nurse-led support prior to surgery and continuity of care. Pulkkinen et al. (2020) advise us that, as a result of the randomisation process, the two groups were found to be similar at baseline and balanced for characteristics such as demographics, type of operation and pre-operative general health status. This is reported in Table 1 of the paper where the numbers in brackets are the percentages, and you can see that these look relatively similar to the naked eye. This is what would be expected after the process of randomisation and many researchers do comment to affirm this or discuss it further in their paper's discussion section if there was a difference at baseline (often stating it as an explanation for finding no difference at the end of the trial).

Table 1 Characteristics of the study participants (*n* = 450)

From: The effect of a new perioperative practice model on length of hospital stay and on the surgical care process in patients undergoing hip and knee arthroplasty under spinal anesthesia: a randomized clinical trial

	Intervention group	Control group	Total
Gender, n (%)			
Male	85 (37.0)	83 (37.7)	168
Female	145 (63.0)	137 (62.3)	282
Age (mean, SD)	67 (10.41)	68 (10.48)	67 (10.44)
Type of operation, n (%)			
THA	143 (62.2)	137 (62.3)	280
TKA	87 (37.8)	83 (37.7)	170
ASA score, n (%)			
ASA 1	30 (13.0)	32 (14.6)	62
ASA2	102 (44.4)	107 (48.6)	209
ASA 3–4	98 (42.6)	81 (36.8)	179

Figure 6.1   Table 1 from Pulkkinen et al. (2020)

Once the outcome measures have been collected at the pre-determined end point for the study, researchers can then compare the results between the groups to ascertain whether there was a difference between the intervention and the control condition. Pulkkinen et al. (2020) present their results in Table 2 of their paper; this table presents both descriptive data (e.g. average length of time) and the statistics that have been applied to help answer the trial question. The descriptive data includes the mean time taken in surgery for the intervention and the control group, for the two types of surgery and by the patients' sex. This is presented in hours and is therefore relatively straightforward to identify. This is followed by a calculation of the difference between the mean for the two groups: intervention and control.

There are two types of analysis that are usually conducted on RCT data: intention to treat analysis (sometimes called 'ITT') and per-protocol analysis. ITT assesses the effect of assigning participants to an intervention, even if they drop out of that group, whereas in per-protocol analysis researchers investigate the effect of what they actually received. The paper (and the protocol) should state which approach is being used. The reason for the two types of analysis is that it is common for people to drop out of a trial or to change groups, and researchers need to know what to do with these patients' data when that occurs. Analysing the data of people who have dropped out of a group as if they are still in their initial group (ITT analysis) may seem counter-intuitive, but it is a way of ensuring that analysis better reflects real life, as not everyone adheres to treatment. Pulkkinen et al. (2020) designed their RCT using per-protocol analysis.

The confidence intervals for the difference in the mean score between the two arms of the study, presented in Table 2 of the paper, indicate what the likely difference in means between the two groups would be if the trial had been undertaken on the whole population of people undergoing total hip or knee arthroplasty. In general terms, the closer the confidence intervals are, the more confident we can be that the results do, in fact, represent the findings if a much larger population was included in the study.

BOX 6.1: CONFIDENCE INTERVALS

Specifically, confidence intervals inform us how confident we should be that 95% of the results fall between the two numbers reported. For example, a CI = 9–11 indicates that we are 95% confident that the results lie between 9–11. However, there is still a 5% risk of chance that they don't.

If we look at the descriptive data first, we can see, for example, that length of stay (bottom of Table 2 in the paper) is reported at 3.08 days for the intervention group and 3.18 days for the controls. The difference between the means is –0.10. This seems very small. The confidence intervals are (–0.40,0.19), indicating that the difference could be larger than –0.10. The confidence intervals provide an estimate of length of stay and are likely to be an accurate reflection of the true population rate within a few hours, as –0.10 falls within this range.

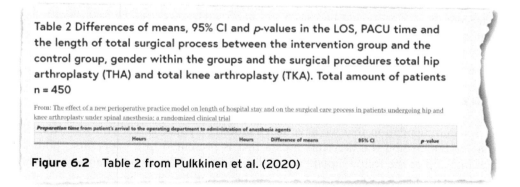

Table 2 Differences of means, 95% CI and *p*-values in the LOS, PACU time and the length of total surgical process between the intervention group and the control group, gender within the groups and the surgical procedures total hip arthroplasty (THA) and total knee arthroplasty (TKA). Total amount of patients n = 450

From: The effect of a new perioperative practice model on length of hospital stay and on the surgical care process in patients undergoing hip and knee arthroplasty under spinal anesthesia: a randomized clinical trial

Figure 6.2 Table 2 from Pulkkinen et al. (2020)

In addition to the descriptive data and confidence intervals provided in Table 2 of the paper, we are also given a p value; this is shown in the final column of the table. This is the result of a statistical test which helps us decide whether a result is likely due to a change that was made or is a result of chance. If there is a true difference between the two groups, the p value will be low: a p value of greater than $p = 0.05$ is generally interpreted to mean that the results could be due to chance, whilst the lower the p value, the less likely the results are due to chance. If we continue to look at Pulkkinen et al.'s (2020) length of stay (reported at the bottom of Table 2 of the paper), we can see that the length of stay was slightly shorter for the intervention group by –0.10 which, when converted into hours, is 2.40 hours. This seems a small amount of time and does not equate to the half day the researchers had hoped they might achieve. Pulkkinen et al. (2020) calculated a p value of 0.49 for the difference in length of stay between those who received the intervention and those who did not. This indicates that the difference in length of stay is likely to be due to chance and so the difference seen in the descriptive data is a statistically non-significant finding. Indeed, when we converted the mean difference into actual hours, we could anticipate that this was unlikely to be significant and the statistical test undertaken confirmed this. Regardless of whether it was statistically significant, you have to think, 'Was it worth it?' Remember that the researchers consider half a day to be a clinically significant difference – do you think it is? It is at this point that we would need to engage the help of a health economist to help us determine whether something that saves a few hours for each patient is an economically, as well as clinically, important intervention.

It is also important to note that just because a trial does not find a statistically significant difference between the results of the intervention and the control group, it does not mean that no difference actually exists. All studies are subject to error, and smaller studies in particular, that do not identify a significant difference between two groups, are subject to type 2 error. This is where the researchers conclude that no difference exists between the groups (as was the case for the length of stay for the participants in the intervention and the control group) when, in reality, a real difference does exist, but the trial's sample size was not large enough to detect this. That is, a larger trial, with greater numbers of patients in the intervention and control groups, might have identified a difference between the groups using the same intervention. We can never be sure if a study is subject to a type 2 error, but it is a concept to keep in mind.

How did they present the results?

One recommendation that we have when reading a paper is that you give yourself time to understand the descriptive data that is presented in a paper first, both at baseline and at the follow-up(s). You will then have a better understanding of who the participants were and what the researchers found as they began to analyse the results. However, this descriptive data alone is not enough for us to fully understand what is happening in a study and this is where we need to draw on additional statistics to help us identify any differences between the groups. For example, in Pulkinnen et al. (2020), Table 2 also presents confidence intervals, which tell us the likely range of results expected if the trial had been conducted on the entire population rather than a sample.

The results are presented in Pulkinnen et al. (2020) as text, in a figure and in tables. As mentioned above, we suggest that you read the full narrative of the paper first to ensure that you understand the flow of numbers throughout the trial: for example, how many participants were in each group, how many dropped out, and so on. Pulkinnen et al. (2020) present this information in a flow diagram in Figure 1 of their paper.

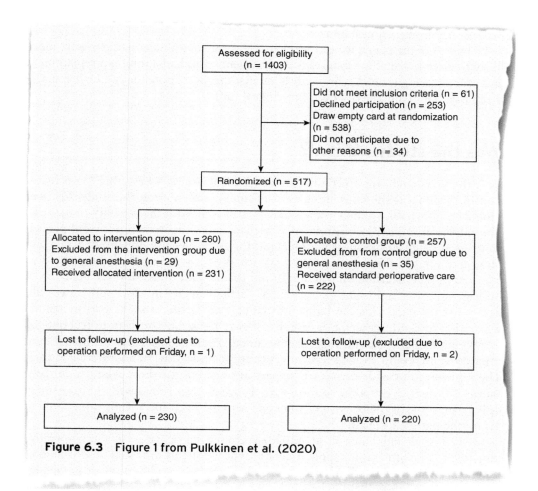

Figure 6.3   Figure 1 from Pulkkinen et al. (2020)

Once you have got an understanding of the descriptive data presented in the paper (e.g. the frequencies in Table 1 of the paper and the mean difference between the groups in Table 2 of the paper), look at how the additional statistics are used to formally test the descriptive data. Table 2 of the paper presented the differences between the groups for all of the outcome measures, including surgery time, operating room time, recovery time and length of stay.

Interestingly, significant differences were found between the intervention and control groups for surgery time and operating room time, but it was the control group who had reduced time (rather than the intervention group) which might have been expected given the nature of the intervention, as the intervention group had the same nurse accompanying them throughout the procedure. The difference between time in surgery was reported at 0.02 and operating room time at 0.01. However, when converted into actual time, the differences for both outcomes was a matter of minutes and not considered to be clinically important (and so of little value clinically). Whilst statistical significance tells us about the reliability of a study's results, clinical significance reflects its likely impact on clinical practice – what real difference it will make in day-to-day clinical practice.

In Table 3 of the paper, we can see that, not surprisingly, older patients were more likely to be in hospital for longer, as were patients who had a total hip replacement and who had a higher ASA score, indicating that they were potentially a higher anaesthetic risk. This could be of interest to clinical staff.

Was the study ethical?

As with all research, the RCT can generate ethical issues. A key ethical consideration in this trial is the consenting of participants on entering the study. Consent should be informed, voluntary and made by someone with the capacity to consent. The information-giving requirement is perhaps most easily met; potential participants must be given full information about the study (what will happen, when and how, and any possible foreseen impacts), usually in writing, which they can then consider in their decision on whether or not to take part. In addition to being given information, it is important that potential participants do not feel under any obligation to take part. This can happen if patients are invited to take part in a study whilst they are still in receipt of care, but it is still possible for them to feel obliged to take part after a period of care has ended. Finally, only those with sufficient capacity can consent to take part in research, or indeed in standard clinical care. The decision to provide care (or take part in research) for those who cannot consent is different in different countries but is usually associated with an assessment of best interests, or the consent of someone who has been specifically nominated to act on the patient's behalf.

In their trial, Pulkkinen et al. (2020) recruited participants at a pre-operative outpatient appointment: an appointment at which patients are likely to be anxious, potentially vulnerable and arguably more likely to feel an obligation to participate rather than risk 'upsetting' the hospital staff. It is not clear whether steps were taken to guard against this. Such steps might include those caring for the patient in a clinical capacity refraining from involvement in the recruitment process, although interestingly ethics committees often request that the researchers do not approach patients directly in order to avoid any suggestion that the patient might feel obliged to participate. Hence, the question of ensuring that potential participants do not feel obliged to participate is a difficult one to manage in clinical practice. However, this trial could be considered a low-risk study, so these considerations are of less concern.

An additional consideration in relation to participant consent to enter a standard RCT is that participants need to be willing to be allocated to either the intervention or the control group; they cannot request a particular group (although some trial designs allow this). Participants consent to be allocated to one treatment or intervention group or another; they have to accept the allocation which is identified at random. Whilst a lot of work is undertaken to ensure that each group is as safe as it can be, and there are steps researchers can take to ensure that any new intervention is as good as standard care, we can never be 100% certain. Questions such as whether it is safe to withhold the usual care or treatment and replace it with an experimental drug or intervention, are significant ones. It is therefore important that potential participants are informed about the evidence for the different interventions before they consent to take part. For Pulkkinen et al.'s study, the intervention cannot be considered high risk, but this is clearly not the case for all studies.

How confident can we be of the results?

The discussion section for this paper provides a debate about what the findings mean for the usefulness of the nursing intervention and the continuity of nursing care for patients undergoing total knee and hip replacement arthroplasty. The study did not show any benefit of the nurse-led intervention as the trial results did not indicate that the intervention had a significant impact on length of stay or other factors associated with surgery. These findings were disappointing for the researchers, given their earlier pilot study. Researchers who plan a study to test their intervention are usually hoping for a positive or significant finding.

It is possible that the design of the study contributed to the lack of significant findings. The study randomised individual patients and if the same nurses provided care for all patients, irrespective of whether they were in the treatment or intervention group, this could have contaminated the standard care that was given to those in the control group. This could be avoided by using a cluster design, where randomisation occurs at a ward or hospital level rather than at the level of the individual patient. In this case, all patients in an intervention ward (or hospital) would have received the intervention and been compared to a ward (or hospital) where all patients received standard or usual care.

It is also important to note that the trial, unlike the pilot study, did not consider the more person-centred and nursing-relevant outcomes such as reduced patient anxiety, satisfaction or preparation for discharge, which might have been improved in those who received the intervention and could therefore have been a significant finding for nursing care; the authors acknowledge this in the paper. This illustrates how the decision researchers make about which outcomes to collect data on (and, in particular, what the primary outcome will be) is therefore very important.

In summary

In this chapter we have summarised what to look for when reading a randomised controlled trial. RCTs are often described as the gold standard of research when we want to find out if something works or not. However, as with all research, it is important to consider whether the design and conduct of the study were optimal as this will affect the quality and usefulness of the evidence it provides. For an RCT, the main quality indicators are whether the sample size was big enough to answer the question, whether allocation into groups was truly random, whether blinding of researchers and participants was possible, whether attrition from the study was minimal and whether the outcomes were appropriate. If these conditions are present in a trial which is large enough to show a difference between the groups, then any differences identified can be reasonably attributed to the intervention rather than chance variation. Pulkinnen et al. (2020) did not identify that nurse-led care led to shorter length of stay – this is an important, if disappointing, finding. It is important because we should not assume that interventions will be effective and RCTs help us to identify those which are and those which are not.

BOX 6.2: QUESTIONS TO ASK YOURSELF ABOUT AN EXPERIMENTAL STUDY

When reading an experimental paper, always ask:

- What was the aim of the trial?
- Was the sample size big enough?
- Were the participants randomised?
- Were the participants and researchers blinded to who received the intervention?
- What proportion dropped out?
- What outcomes were measured?
- Were the differences between the groups statistically significant?

NOTE

We were able to make contact with Maria Pulkkinen, the lead author of this paper: Maria was delighted to share her paper in this book and did not add further comment.

SUGGESTED READING

Schultz, K. and Grimes, D. (2018) *Essential Concepts in Clinical Research: Randomised Controlled Trials and Observational Studies* (2nd edition). Oxford: Elsevier.

7 A case-control study paper

In the previous chapter, we focused on the design of a randomised controlled trial (RCT): a design which is highly controlled and used to compare the effectiveness of an intervention or treatment for those who received it with those who did not. In an RCT, any difference in outcomes can be reasonably attributed to the intervention if the trial design was sufficiently adhered to. The majority of researchers agree that the RCT is the only true way to establish the effectiveness of an intervention and is therefore a design that is of fundamental importance in scientific enquiry and health care. However, designing a study with such a high level of control is not always possible, nor even appropriate or desirable. The design of a study should always map, or reflect, the research question. Some possible deviations from the design of a traditional RCT are mentioned in the previous chapter – for example, where a new service is being developed and strict individual randomisation (e.g. where an individual patient is randomised) would be difficult. In this case, cluster randomisation can instead be used (where randomisation occurs at a higher level, such as in a ward, hospital or GP practice with another service acting as the control). Where randomisation itself is not possible, a simple before-and-after design can be used to test an intervention. This is a much weaker design as, without the randomisation, we cannot be as confident that the findings are due to the intervention rather than other factors that may vary between those who get the intervention and those who do not. Studies which deviate from the controlled design of the RCT, such as a case-controlled study, are often referred to as quasi-experiments: there are many designs for these, and it is beyond the scope of this book to discuss all possible variations, but we will explore one in this chapter.

A case-control study is not a form of experiment, hence it is referred to as a 'quasi-experiment'. It is a quantitative, observational study designed to help determine if an exposure to something (for example, smoking or pollen) is associated with an increased likelihood of a certain outcome (for example a disease, a condition or an event). There are two groups within a case-control study: the cases (where the event happened) and the controls (where it did not). So, you can see some similarities with an experiment (or RCT), but in a case-control study the groups are naturally occurring: they are not created as part of the research design and participants are not 'allocated' to them – they are already there. Case-control studies enable the researcher to identify the likely causes of an outcome that is present in one group but not in the other, and where it is possible to look back and see what factors were also present only in the group in which the outcome occurred.

The 'cases' are participants who have a condition or who have experienced an event that researchers are interested in the causes of. The 'controls' are participants who are similar to the cases but do not have the particular condition or have not had the experience of the event of interest. Researchers then compare factors that are (or are not) present in the cases and controls in order to identify possible causes of the condition or event. These studies are predominantly epidemiological studies and are used to explore the relationship between the risk and the occurrence of certain events; for example, this study design was famously used to identify the link between smoking and lung cancer in the 1960s. In a series of case-control studies, the possible risk factors of those who developed lung cancer were examined and compared with a similar group of people who did not develop lung cancer (Cicco et al., 2016). Through this approach, smoking was identified as the key risk factor. Where researchers seek to establish a link between two variables, rather than establishing the effectiveness of an intervention on those groups, then a case-control study could be an appropriate design.

Another type of quantitative observational study is a cohort study. Cohort studies explore the relationship between factors from a longitudinal perspective, following up a group or cohort of people over time to see what risk factors lead to which diseases or outcomes. Cohort studies are usually, but not exclusively, prospective, whereas case-control studies are usually, but not exclusively, retrospective: the key difference is that there are no controls in cohort studies. Cohort designs were also used for the early studies undertaken to explore the risk factors for lung cancer: those who smoked were followed up and the incidence of lung cancer in those who smoked was compared to those who did not smoke (Cicco et al., 2016). Whilst both case-control studies and cohort studies are often used within epidemiology, these designs can also be used in the clinical environment.

The case-control study we will explore in this chapter is:

de Groot, G. C. L., Al-Fattal, A. and Sandven, I. (2020) Falls in hospital: A case-control study. *Scandinavian Journal of Caring Sciences*, 34: 332–9.

Get yourself a copy of the paper, read it through, then work/read through the rest of the chapter, finding the points we identify in the paper: https://onlinelibrary.wiley.com/doi/epdf/10.1111/scs.12733

Scan the QR code to be taken straight to the paper.

What does the abstract and information about the authors tell me?

In this abstract, the aim is a bit confusing as it includes some background information, so you may need to read the introduction of the main body of the paper to really understand it. However, from the aim in the main body of the paper, it is clear that the researchers are 'investigating the major risk factors for falls in the hospital setting'.

From the abstract, we can see that the paper reports on a retrospective case-control study of 842 patients, 172 of whom had experienced a fall during their hospital admission. Retrospective means looking backwards rather than forwards. The 670 controls had not fallen during their hospital admission. Possible risk factors were identified from the literature and previous pilot work, and these risk factors were then looked for in those who had experienced a fall and those who had not. The abstract also summarises the main findings and conclusions.

FALLS IN HOSPITAL: A CASE-CONTROL STUDY

Aims:

Falls among inpatients are common. The method used by The Norwegian Patient Safety Campaign to measure the adverse events is the Global Trigger Tool, which does not look at the causation for falls. This study was aimed at investigating major risk factors for falls in the hospital setting.

Methods:

This retrospective case-control study was conducted at Telemark Hospital in Norway, in the period from September 2012 to August 2014. A total of 842 patients from three wards were included, whereof 172 cases had experienced one or more fall(s) during hospitalisation and 670 random controls had not fallen. Data was analysed according to a pragmatic strategy.

Results:

Compared with patients who did not fall, patients who fell were 21 times more likely to have poor balance (OR = 21.50, 95% CI: 10.26–45.04) and 19 times more likely to have very poor balance (OR = 19.62, 95% CI: 9.55–40.27), twice as likely to be men (OR = 1.82, 95% CI: 1.24–2.68), and [having a] 50% increased probability of fall with every 10-year increase of age (OR = 1.51, 95% CI: 1.34–1.69). Furthermore, the patients who fell were more likely to use antidepressant drugs (OR = 3.85, 95% CI: 1.09–13.63), antipsychotic drugs (OR = 3.27, 95% CI: 1.94–5.51), anxiolytic/hypnotic drugs (OR = 1.80, 95% CI: 1.22–2.67) and antiepileptic drugs (OR = 1.13, 95% CI: 1.11–4.06) than patients who did not fall.

Conclusions:

During hospital stay, patients who fell had a higher risk profile than patients who did not fall. Clinicians should work to improve patients' safety and reduce

(Continued)

the risk of falls by accurately assessing balance and mobility as a form of primary prevention. We recommend that a review of the patient medications should be conducted upon falling, as a form of a secondary preventative strategy against falls.

Keywords: Antidepressants, Balance, Drugs, Falls, Hospital

We are told in the paper that the authors include a physical therapist, a physician and a PhD student (so we can probably assume from this that the study was undertaken as part of a doctoral programme) at the Oslo Centre of Biostatistics and Epidemiology, with the support of academic supervisors from the Telemark Hospital in Norway.

Is there a clear research question or aim addressed by the research?

This study used an aim rather than a research question. The aim of the study is clear within the main body of the paper: to investigate major risk factors for falls in the hospital setting. The rationale for this was that identifying risk factors could reduce the incidence of falls in hospital. We are told that the hospital had been identified as a pilot site for a patient safety project. This study aim is clearly useful given the importance of preventing falls within hospital, and understanding their cause could help to prevent them if those causes (risk factors) are addressed.

How was the study designed?

Case-control studies are observational studies: that means we look to see what naturally happens or happened (rather than manipulating what happens in any way). In a case-control study, researchers compare 'cases' (who are identified as those who have experienced the phenomenon of interest in the study, in this case patients who had experienced a fall in hospital) and compare these with 'controls' (in this case patients who had not experienced a fall in hospital). Given the comparison element of this study, it is easy to confuse the design with the randomised controlled trial; however, the difference is that researchers are not looking for evidence of effectiveness of a treatment or intervention, and crucially there is no random allocation of participants into groups. Instead, the design enables researchers to examine the circumstances, events, exposure and personal history of the patients who are 'cases' and to compare these to those who are 'controls', in order to determine whether there are factors that are more common in the cases that could then be described as causal, or in the control group that could be described as protective.

De Groot et al. (2020) identified 172 patients who had fallen in hospital within the timeframe of the study. These patients make up the 'cases' in the study. The researchers clearly define how they categorised a fall, emphasising that it did not necessitate incurring an injury.

> Fall was defined as 'an event resulting in a person coming to rest inadvertently on the ground, floor or other lower level, whether there is any damage caused by the fall' (7).

In a case-control study, there are often many potential controls; the controls can be anyone who is similar to the case but who does not have the condition experienced by the case. De Groot et al. (2020) chose to randomly identify 670 'non fallers' from the remaining patients who had been in hospital within this timeframe. This random identification is not the same as random allocation as this study design does not allocate participants to an intervention: it is just a way of finding controls for a study where the number of people not experiencing the condition is much higher than those who have experienced it. It is not necessarily common practice to identify the controls at random from the available controls, but, in the case of de Groot et al. (2020), data about possible risk factors was collected from the notes, so a random sample of controls was a practical option. It is important to note that obtaining a random sample of controls does not mean that the characteristics of participants in the case and control groups are equally distributed and that the groups are essentially matched as in a randomised controlled trial, but it takes out the element of selection and potential bias from the identification of controls. De Groot et al. (2020) identified one case to every four controls within the study. It is common practice to identify more controls than cases in a case-control study as this adds power to the study, improving the efficiency of statistical analysis.

With the cases and controls established, the aim of the research is to identify whether there were any significant differences between the cases and controls (for example, type of exposure, age) which might account for the outcome under investigation, in this case the incidence of falls in hospital.

What is assessed in a case-control study?

In a case-control study, the *possible* factors that might increase the patients' risk of the outcome of interest are predetermined by the researchers. That is, the researchers make an educated guess, based on previous studies, as to what the potential risk factors *might* be; for instance, those that they want to find out more about and that will be looked for and analysed in the study.

De Groot et al. (2020) identified that age, illness, health status, balance and gender might be contributing factors to falling. However, they did not know this for sure and so, in order to find out, they assessed these factors in both groups – that is, in patients who had fallen and in the controls. In the subsequent analysis, these factors were compared between the groups in order to find out whether, in fact, there was a difference in the incidence of these factors in the cases and controls. Where there is a significant difference of the incidence of a factor between the cases and controls, a risk factor might reasonably be said to have been identified. Where no such difference is identified and the incidence in the cases and the controls is very similar, the factor investigated would not be considered a risk factor.

Are the assessments made available to the reader?

It is standard practice for a list of the assessments to be made available to the reader. The Materials and Methods section of the paper describes the sources of data relating to the predetermined factors the researchers were looking for. Table 2 of the paper lists these possible risk factors alongside the data for each factor analysed.

Who was invited to participate in the study?

The study included patients who had experienced a fall and those who had not, from among past inpatients in one of three wards at a hospital in Norway. These patients did not participate in person however, instead their data was extracted from their medical and nursing notes for analysis. The implications of this are discussed in the next section.

A retrospective case-control study was conducted at Telemark Hospital in Norway. Eligible for inclusion were adults, 18 years or older, admitted to the hospital from September 2012 to August 2014. Participants were recruited from three wards: Neurology, Respiratory medicine and Acute Geriatric medicine.

How did they analyse the results?

The results in a case-control study are analysed by comparing the incidence or prevalence of the predetermined factors (or variables) in the cases and in the controls, in order to find out if there are significant differences in these factors (or variables) between the two groups. From the descriptive data, we can see how often the factors that were being investigated as a possible cause of falls in hospital were present in the cases (those who had fallen) and the controls (those who had not fallen).

It is important to remember that there were four times as many controls as cases when looking at the descriptive data: it can be more meaningful to look at the percentages than the actual numbers. This descriptive data gives us an idea as to possible risk factors for falling – that is, those risk factors that appeared more often in the cases such as use of medication, older age and being male. However, this descriptive data alone is not enough for us to fully understand if there is a statistical difference between the two groups; that is, a difference that is unlikely to be due to chance. As discussed in the previous chapter, this is where we draw on additional statistics to help us identify any real differences between the groups, or whether the differences identified are due to chance.

The statistics used by de Groot et al. (2020) include logistic regression, odds ratios and p values – these were used to calculate whether there was a true difference in the incidence or prevalence (see Box 7.1) of the different factors that might lead to falls between the cases and controls, or whether these differences were due to chance. These can be quite complex statistical terms to understand without further tuition, and detailed understanding is not expected at undergraduate-level study. What is important is that you can interpret what the statistics tell you about the results of the study and, most importantly, what this might mean for clinical practice.

BOX 7.1: INCIDENCE AND PREVALENCE

Note the difference between incidence and prevalence:

- Incidence is the number of newly diagnosed people with a condition;
- Prevalence is the number of people living with a condition across a timespan.

Odds ratios present the odds of a risk affecting the outcome that the researchers are interested in. In this case, odds ratios were used to illustrate what the chances are of having a fall when a certain factor is present. An odds ratio of 1 indicates no difference in the risk; an odds ratio greater than 1 indicates an increased risk. De Groot et al. (2020) compared the prevalence of the pre-identified factors (such as age, sex, health status) in the cases and controls, and calculated odds ratios to identify when these factors increased the odds or chances of a fall; i.e. they looked for an odds ratio of more than 1.

The association between potential risk factors and falls was quantified by the odds ratio (OR) and its 95% confidence interval (CI).

Table 3 of the paper presents those risks that had an odds ratio greater than 1. The odds ratios are accompanied by a confidence interval. Confidence intervals were discussed in the previous chapter and represent the confidence we have that

95% of the findings (i.e. the level of risk of falling) lie between the numbers expressed in the confidence interval. Crucially, therefore, for a risk to be considered more significant in those who had fallen, the odds ratio needs to be greater than 1, but also the range of the numbers in the confidence interval needs to be as close to the odds ratio as possible.

Table 3 Risk factors differentiating patients with fall versus no fall using the multivariate logistic model

Risk factors	Level	OR (95% CI)	p-Value
Model A			
Male sex	Yes/no	1.82 (1.24–2.68)	0.002
Balance	Good	(reference)	
	Poor	21.50 (10.26–45.04)	0.001
	Very poor	19.62 (9.55–40.27)	0.001
Anxiolytics/Hypnotic drugs	Yes/no	1.80 (1.22–2.67)	0.003
Antiepileptic drugs	Yes/no	1.13 (1.11–4.06)	0.022
Antipsychotic drugs	Yes/no	2.01 (1.15–3.51)	0.014
Model B			
Age	10 year increase	1.51 (1.34–1.69)	0.001
Antipsychotic drugs	Yes/no	3.27 (1.94–5.51)	0.001
Antidepressants	Yes/no	3.85 (1.09–13.63)	0.037

CI, confidence interval; OR, odds ratio.
Two-model presentation was used to avoid the problem of collinearity between the risk factors of fall

Figure 7.1   Table 3 from de Groot et al. (2020)

Odds ratios tell us whether there are increased risk factors in one group or another. They do not tell us whether the increased risk is statistically significant. In order to find this out, de Groot et al. (2020) conducted an additional statistical test. Whether or not the difference in risk factors between the case and the control groups were significant is determined by the p value: a statistical concept which was discussed in the previous chapter. The p value is the result of a test which allows us to determine whether a result is due to chance or whether there is a genuine difference between the two groups. A low p value is indicative of a difference that is less likely to be due to chance and therefore more likely to indicate a genuine difference between the two groups. P values are tricky because they don't prove something but just give you the likelihood that a result is (or is not) due to chance. Sometimes we might be confident with a 5% possibility of chance (i.e. a p value of 0.05) but, at other times, you might want less chance of risk for a procedure, for instance a 1% possibility of chance (i.e. a p value of 0.001).

De Groot et al. (2020) found a range of results, some of which were statistically significant and others where the p value did not reach significance, i.e. the p value was more than 0.05. These are discussed in the next section. Rather than just looking at single factors that might influence whether someone falls or not, the researchers grouped risk factors into two models – Model A and Model B. This is important because some risk factors are linked, such as age and poor mobility. You wouldn't want to use them both in the same model as they might inflate the results – this is what they meant when they stated that they wanted to avoid 'collinearity'. Model A included sex and balance and Model B just included age.

How did they present the results?

De Groot et al. (2020) present their results in three tables and provide an accompanying narrative. Table 1 of the paper presents the clinical profile of patients who had fallen and those who had not. In this table, the descriptive data are presented together with the odds ratio, confidence interval and accompanying p value. We can see that there are significant differences for all of the factors listed, including increasing age, being male, having poor balance, having multiple diseases and use of medication, except for those with renal function problems and who use anti-depressants. Table 2 of the paper shows the results of the different age groups and associated risk factors, and Table 3 of the paper shows a further analysis to determine the relationship between the risk factors and the risk of falling, and clearly indicates the risk factors of age, sex, balance and certain drugs that increase the risk of falls.

There are some tricky statistical concepts in this paper. It is not necessary for you to understand these in-depth, but it is useful to have a working understanding of what they mean – how you should interpret them. We have provided an introduction to understanding the statistics but left aside more complicated issues, given that this is an introduction to understanding this type of research paper. The key is to understand the general principles of the statistics and to follow the written narrative. In the previous chapter, we mentioned how important it is to look at the descriptive data (the summary of the raw data) from the study so that you develop an understanding of the sample and the data before any statistical tests are applied. This enables a better understanding of the ultimate results and their interpretation. The following narrative extract from the paper gives an overview of the findings:

Model A shows that the patients who fell had 21 times (OR = 21.50, 95% CI: 10.26–45.04) the prevalence of poor balance and 19 times (OR = 19.62, 95% CI:9.55–40.27) the prevalence of very poor balance as compared to the patients who did not fall. Furthermore, this group was twice as likely to consist of men (OR = 1.82,95% CI: 1.24–2.68), and using/receiving the following drugs: anxiolytic/hypnotic drugs (OR = 1.80, 95% CI:1.22–2.67), antiepileptic drugs (OR = 1.13, 95% CI:1.11–4.06) and antipsychotic drugs (OR = 2.01, 95% CI:1.15–3.51). Model B informs us that the probability of falling increased by 50% with every 10-year increase of age (OR = 1.51, 95% CI: 1.34–1.69). Furthermore, the patients who fell used three times more antipsychotics (OR = 3.27, 95% CI: 1.94–5.51) and antidepressant drugs (OR = 3.85, 95% CI: 1.09–13.63) than the patients who did not fall.

Was the study ethical?

A key ethical consideration in this study is the consent of participants. Consent should be informed, voluntary and made by someone with the capacity to consent. The ethical question for this study is whether consent should be sought prior to extracting data from a patient's notes, even though the patient might never be aware of the study and possibly not even identifiable from the notes. The answer to this will depend in part on the country in which the study is taking place. Different countries interpret the ethical requirements for consent in different ways. If the notes are made truly anonymous, then the requirement for consent from the patient will be less (or even not required). However, other legislation, such as that concerning data protection, has specific requirements about the use of patient data, regardless of whether the patient can be identified from it. De Groot et al. (2020) provided the following statement about ethical approval for the study (it is also not clear whether this required them to obtain the consent of each patient before accessing and analysing the information in their medical records):

> **ETHICAL APPROVAL**
>
> This study was registered at the Norwegian Social Science Data Services (NSD) on 3 June 2015, with the registration number 43162. Enrolment of patients started in February 2016. No ethical approval typical for empirical studies was needed.

It is interesting that they named the hospital within the paper too. Once again, this differs according to ethical requirements as, by naming the site, it potentially leads to the risk of revealing who the individual participants in the study were.

How confident can we be of the results of the study?

The study provides some useful significant results about the risk factors for falls in hospital. These findings are clinically useful and give an element of certainty to risks that might have been predicted but for which there was no specific evidence. As a result, nurses and other clinical staff are advised to do a risk assessment on patient mobility and to review patients' medication in assessing their risk of falling. In this way, patients who are at a risk of falling can be pre-identified and monitored. The researchers also note the limitations of doing research that is reliant on patient documentation, and suggest that more prospective studies are needed – that is, studies collecting data in real time (looking forward), rather than looking back and collecting information from medical notes which might be missing.

In summary

In this chapter we have summarised what to look for when you are reading a case-control study. Case-control studies are usually considered to be lower-quality evidence than RCTs because they rely on naturally occurring data, rather than actively recruiting patients and randomising them to a control or an intervention group. They are therefore less controlled and more susceptible to bias. However, it is often not possible to use formally controlled study designs, and case-control studies can provide useful data despite the increased risk of bias that is inherent in them. Case-control studies explore risk factors that might lead to adverse events (such as falls) and compare these with the same possible risk factors in (natural) controls who did not have the adverse event. Although they involve the comparison of different groups, they are not always strong evidence due to the fact that these groups are not created at random. This is the main limitation in the study design. However, case-control studies provide useful data and a great understanding of the risk factors for adverse events and diseases, and therefore often provide useful data for understanding the causes of such events.

BOX 7.2: QUESTIONS TO ASK YOURSELF ABOUT A CASE-CONTROL STUDY

When reading a case-control study paper, always ask:

- How was the study designed?
- Where were the data collected from?
- How many were in the sample?
- What risk factors or variables were investigated and why?
- How were the data analysed?
- How confident do you feel in the results?

NOTE

We were unable to make contact with the authors of this paper.

SUGGESTED READING

Schultz, K. and Grimes, D. (2018) *Essential Concepts in Clinical Research: Randomised Controlled Trials and Observational Studies* (2nd edition). Oxford: Elsevier.

8 A mixed methods study paper

So far in this book, we have discussed individual methods for addressing research questions. We have examined qualitative approaches and we have examined quantitative approaches. Qualitative methods are generally used when we want to explore people's experiences and perceptions, and quantitative methods are generally used when we are seeking numerical measurement and possibly looking for relationships between different variables (for example, mental health and working hours) by applying statistical tests in order to test the link between them and the generalisability of the findings. Whether a qualitative or quantitative approach is used depends entirely on the research question or aim of the study; it is usually fairly intuitive which approach will have been used when you look at the title or research question in a paper – although, of course, not always.

If we think back to the papers we have appraised within this book, you can see how the different research questions were addressed by different methods and approaches, some of them qualitative and some of them quantitative:

- The mental health of nurses was examined in a survey of hospital staff using pre-tested questionnaires that the researchers were confident would measure mental health in a valid and reliable way (Chapter 2: Surveys – quantitative).
- The way in which nurses assess and manage depression in older patients was examined qualitatively using in-depth interviews as little was known about this topic (Chapter 3: Qualitative research – no specific method).
- The meaning of good surgical care was explored through a specific qualitative research method known as grounded theory as the researchers wanted to identify a theory or model to explain good care (Chapter 4: Grounded theory – qualitative).

- Patients' and carers' experience of chronic obstructive pulmonary disease was explored through phenomenology, which is a qualitative method specifically used for the study of the meaning of experiences (Chapter 5: Phenomenology – qualitative).
- Whether or not a new approach to peri-operative care reduced the time spent in hospital was investigated in an experiment, known as a randomised controlled trial (RCT). In an RCT, researchers want to find out if there is a difference in the outcome between groups which is caused by their intervention (Chapter 6: Randomised controlled trial – quantitative).
- The causes of falls in hospital were examined using a case-control study, which is a quasi-experimental observational study. In this study, the risk factors for falls were carefully compared among those who had had falls and those who had not (Chapter 7: Case-control study – quantitative).

All of these studies used an appropriate method to collect data in order to answer their research question or study aim. Researchers undertaking exploratory studies used a qualitative approach and method, and researchers whose aim was to measure numerically (and test for associations) used a quantitative approach and method. However, in all of the studies, we could see limitations in the approach used: qualitative studies cannot be generalised and quantitative studies can lack insight into details that could be provided by a more qualitative approach, such as why something happens or how it happens (rather than whether it happens or how often). A solution to this is to combine qualitative and quantitative approaches to provide more comprehensive, rounded answers on a topic. This is the purpose of mixed methods research: researchers use both qualitative and quantitative methods to answer a single or set of research questions or aims, using the merits of each approach to shed light on the question(s), using both types of data, where appropriate. It is beyond the scope or requirements of many projects to take a mixed methods approach – and such an approach may not always be appropriate; however, this approach is becoming increasingly popular in health care as, if done well, it can provide a better understanding of health care problems than either approach alone.

There are many different mixed methods study designs. They are typically named according to the order in which the two types of approaches (quantitative and qualitative) are used and their goal. Creswell and Plano Clark (2011) describe three main types of mixed methods study design:

- Convergent design: where the qualitative and quantitative components take place simultaneously.
- Explanatory sequential design: where the quantitative study is undertaken first, and the subsequent qualitative study is conducted to explore and explain the findings of the quantitative study.
- Exploratory sequential design: where the qualitative study is undertaken first and subsequent quantitative research is conducted to confirm, or establish, the commonality of issues identified in the qualitative study.

There are many more mixed methods designs, but these three are the most common. A mixed methods approach can therefore occur within a single study or across a programme of work made up of several studies.

The key thing to remember, and to look for in a mixed methods study, is an integration of the two approaches (Bazeley, 2009). At some point, the two approaches should 'speak' to each other; they should be integrated, and this should happen before the researchers draw any conclusions from the study. Also, the integrated findings should be greater than the sum of the parts: this means that the end product of a mixed methods study (the conclusion) should be something that would not have been available without that integration. This integration can happen at different stages of the research process: where and how much it occurs will vary by study, depending on the aims or research question(s). For example, it can occur within the study design (where analysis of quantitative survey findings identifies a set of issues for exploration in a sub-sample of participants by qualitative methods), it can occur during analysis (where the two types of data are brought together for analysis, or one informs how the other is analysed), or it can happen after data has been collected and the two approaches have been analysed separately (where the two sets of findings are compared or used to interpret one another). There are different, well-established techniques for doing this and O'Cathain et al. (2010) provide a useful introduction to these.

A mixed methods study is not a study that simply collects only multiple types of qualitative data, or only multiple types of quantitative data – these types of studies are usually called 'multi-method studies'. And studies that do collect both types of data (quantitative and qualitative) but do not integrate them at any point are technically not mixed methods studies (even though they often use this label). As we have seen before in this book, the terminology used in research – as with terminology used in many aspects of life – is not always consistent.

When we are reading a mixed methods study, all of our knowledge and understanding of the separate approaches and methods (quantitative and qualitative) remain important, but we should also look for that integration of the two approaches that is so important in mixed methods work.

The mixed methods paper we will explore in this chapter is:

Dousin, O., Collins, N., Bartram, T. and Stanton, P. (2021) The relationship between work–life balance, the need for achievement, and intention to leave: Mixed-method study. *Journal of Advanced Nursing*, 77: 1478–89.

Get yourself a copy of the paper, read it through, then work/read through the rest of the chapter, finding the points we identify in the paper: https://onlinelibrary.wiley.com/doi/epdf/10.1111/jan.14724

Scan the QR code to be taken straight to the paper.

What does the abstract and information about the authors tell me?

The abstract should be a concise account of the study that provides enough information to enable you to assess whether to access the paper in full. We are told that the paper is a mixed methods study (this is also stated in the title), conducting a quantitative questionnaire/survey followed by qualitative interviews. This is an explanatory design, enabling the researchers to follow up on the findings of the written survey in in-depth interviews. The abstract therefore describes the study design as an explanatory mixed methods design. The focus of the study is to examine the work–life balance of nurses in Malaysia.

ABSTRACT

Aims

To examine the mediating role of employee well-being on the relationship between work–life balance practices, the need for achievement and intention to leave among nurses in Malaysia.

Background

Work–life balance practices are associated with employee perceptions of the need for achievement and well-being which subsequently influence their intention to leave the organisation. This study contributes new knowledge to nursing studies on work–life balance in an Asian and Islamic society where the expectations for women are to focus on family rather than career.

Design

A cross-sectional, explanatory mixed methodology.

Methods

This is a two-phase study conducted between 2015–2017 with 401 nurses in East Malaysia. In Phase 1, researchers surveyed 379 nurses to test eight hypotheses and in Phase 2 researchers interviewed 22 nurses to explore the results of Phase 1.

Results

Phase 1 revealed job satisfaction mediates the relationship between work–life balance practices (e.g. flexibility and choice in working hours, supportive supervision), financial success, and intention to leave. However, life satisfaction and money as a motivator did not mediate such relationships. Phase 2 identified four important factors that cast light on survey results: working conditions of Malaysian nurses; inadequate compensation in the public health care sector; team-based practices; and pressure on senior nurses in both administrative and clinical roles.

Conclusion

This is one of the first studies to investigate work–life balance issues among nurses in Malaysia. Outcomes of this study extend the debates on work–life balance and employee well-being in an Asian Islamic social context.

Impact

The use of flexible working arrangements and collectivist teamwork approaches, improving compensation and employment benefits and eliminating the 'time-based job promotion' policy, may help to mitigate work–life balance issues and intention to leave among nurses in Malaysia.

Interestingly, this abstract doesn't just end with a 'Conclusion' section, but also has an 'Impact' section. Increasingly, researchers are being challenged to report what the impact of their research might be. Health care research might suggest a change in practice or, as in the case of this study, a change in policy relating to flexible working arrangements. This is the 'so what' element of research – 'so why does the research you are reading matter?' or 'what difference does this make?'.

The study was undertaken in Malaysia, with the support of colleagues in Australia. We are not told the background of the researchers, but we can see that they hold academic positions in faculties of business and economics (rather than health or health care).

Is there a clear research question or aim addressed by the research?

In their introduction, the authors discuss the pressures on the nursing workforce in Malaysia, the national nursing shortage, the cultural context and the possibilities of working abroad and attaining a higher salary. Hence, many nurses experience a pull to leave Malaysia. The geographical area in which the study was undertaken is described as an area experiencing high nurse attrition to work in other areas; the need to improve staff retainment is clear. The researchers suggest that one way to improve the retainment of staff is to improve the work–life balance of the workforce; their mixed methods study therefore sought to investigate this. In view of this, the research question was: *Does nurse well-being mediate the relationships between work–life balance, the need for achievement and intention to leave; if so, why?* The research question is a little hidden in the introduction, although the researchers have a clear aim in the abstract and also in the main part of the paper (under the heading 'Aims').

The research question is: does nurse well-being mediate the relationships between WLB, the need for achievement and intention to leave; if so, why?

2.1 AIMS

The study examines the mediating role of employee well-being on the relation-ship between work–life balance (WLB) practices, the need for achievement and intention to leave among nurses in Malaysia. Evidence suggests the WLB practices assist employees to attain their personal and professional goals and those who experience WLB practices report greater well-being and more posi-tive role-specific experience, leading to an increase in motivation, commitment, and reducing intention to leave.

The researchers also state eight hypotheses to test in the study. A hypothesis is a state-ment of an expected outcome which researchers either go on to prove or disprove through the study, as discussed in Chapter 6. The use of a hypothesis in research is only relevant in quantitative research where it can be tested using numerical measures. In this study, Dousin et al. (2021) state that, for example, their hypothesis 1 that 'Job satisfaction will mediate the relationship between flexibility and choice in working hours and intention to leave'. They planned to use the quantitative data from the survey to find support for this hypothesis. As we have seen in previous chapters relating to quantitative study designs, not all quantitative research questions are accompanied by a hypothesis; similarly, not all quantitative components of mixed methods studies include them.

How was the study designed?

Dousin et al. (2021) described their study as using an explanatory mixed methods design – given that they describe collecting and analysing quantitative data (through a survey), then qualitative data (through follow-up interviews), we could extend this label to an explanatory *sequential* mixed methods design. This design can be used when there is sufficient knowledge about the topic being researched to develop a survey or questionnaire, or where a pre-existing questionnaire or outcome measure is available. Where less is known about a topic, qualitative interviews might be used initially in order to develop a questionnaire or outcome measure – this would be described as an *exploratory* sequential mixed methods design.

The study had two phases. Phase 1 was the quantitative survey, designed to gain an understanding of Malaysian nurses' work–life balance practices, need for achievement, and well-being and intention to leave. This was followed by Phase 2, the qualitative interview study with nurses, to further explore and cast light on the results of the Phase 1 survey, through in-depth exploration of their opinions based on their own experiences. From this, we can see that Dousin et al. (2021) were using both quantitative and qualitative methods of data collection and analysis, and using the former to inform the latter in order to more fully understand the issues around work–life balance for nurses in Malaysia.

2.2 DESIGN

This study adopts a cross-sectional, explanatory mixed-methods two-phased approach. Phase 1 was a quantitative survey conducted between October and December 2015, followed by phase 2, qualitative in-depth interviews with nurses conducted between December 2016 and February 2017.

Looking at the two phases in more detail, in Phase 1, Dousin et al. (2021) undertook a survey on a sample of nurses who worked in a region of Malaysia in which there was a high turnover of staff. In Chapter 2, we discussed research that uses questionnaires and surveys. Dousin et al. (2021) used a convenience sample of hospitals within two geographically remote states with poorer infrastructure than the rest of Malaysia – the rationale for this being that nurses in these states faced high work demands. Hospitals from city, rural and remote areas were selected, from which nurses were invited to participate. It is tricky to find this information in the paper, as you might expect it to be included in section 2.3 where they describe the sample, but instead it is in a section entitled '2.4 Data collection'.

2.4 DATA COLLECTION

In 2017, there were 43 public hospitals and 16 private hospitals in Sabah and Sarawak. The study took place in six public hospitals and three private hospitals in these states. Convenience sampling (Sekaran and Bougie, 2013) was adopted and hospitals from city, rural, and remote areas were selected.

The researchers used a standard table created by Krejcie and Morgan (1970) to calculate the sample size. As stated in Chapter 2, researchers need a representative sample for a survey, especially when the population of interest is very large. Krejcie and Morgan (1970) developed a calculation to identify representative sample sizes for different populations. Dousin et al. (2021) knew the number of nurses in these regions was 20,305 and, by using Krejcie and Morgan's (1970) table, they calculated that they needed a sample size of 377 to be representative of this population. In order to achieve this sample of 377 nurses, the researchers sent out questionnaires to 388 nurses – this did not give much leeway for non-responders, and they did not give a rationale for this number. In fact, they received 379 completed questionnaires, which represents a response rate of 97.7%. As discussed in Chapter 2, response rates to surveys can be very low and so this is a very high response rate and suggests that the researchers had a highly controlled method for distributing and ensuring the return of completed questionnaires. We could speculate that the nurses perhaps completed the questionnaires at the start of a shift and handed them back immediately on completion.

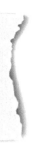

According to the Department of Statistics Malaysia (2019, 2020), the number of nurses in Sabah and Sarawak in 2017 was 20,305. Following Krejcie and Morgan's (1970) sample size determination, for a population of 20,000, a sample size of 377 was deemed adequate. A total of 388 surveys were distributed and participants returned their completed questionnaires in a confidential envelope to the Chief Investigator. Cases with missing data for the key variables were deleted, resulting in a final sample of 379 nurses (97.7% response rate).

We also discussed in Chapter 2 the importance of the use of a well-constructed questionnaire within a survey. Ideally, researchers should give details of the questionnaire, whether it has been tested for use with the population of interest or used before in other (similar) studies. Dousin et al. (2021) do provide some information on this but, again, do so in an unusual place in the paper; we would normally expect to see this information reported in the methods section but unusually, they provide this detail at the start of the results section – you can find it under the heading 'Measures' (section 3.1.1, page 1482). Here, they reported that they used the 7-point Likert scale (described in Table 2.1, Chapter 2), ranging from 'strongly disagree/dissatisfied', which is given a rank of 1, to 'strongly agree/satisfied', which is given a rank of 7, to measure a series of components relating to work–life balance practices, need for achievement, employee well-being, and intention to leave. They used some established scales for doing this such as the 'Love of Money' Scale (Tang and Chiu, 2003). We are told that the questionnaires were adapted for use in the current study, but little detail on this adaptation is given. This adaptation may have been to make them more culturally acceptable, but in general we use questionnaires as they were developed in order to ensure retention of their validity and reliability. Often, questionnaires undergo some sort of testing to adapt them to other cultures and it looks like the 'Love of Money' Scale was tested in other cultural groups prior to use in this study.

When multiple questionnaires are used to measure the same issue, tests can be completed to see how the results correlate with one another. The researchers used a test called the Cronbach Alpha where the closer the value is to one, the greater the level of correlation. You don't need to understand too much about these tests, but it is helpful to understand that a correlation suggests that there is a relationship between the factors or variables. However, do beware of spurious correlations: these occur where a mathematical relationship is found between two or more factors, suggesting that they are associated when they are not actually causally related. This can occur due to either coincidence or the presence of a third, unseen factor. Correlations should make some sort of logical sense. There is a fun website you can explore that gives real-world examples of spurious correlations: www.tylervigen.com/spurious-correlations

For Phase 2, Dousin et al. (2021) undertook qualitative interviews with a subset of nurses who had completed the questionnaire. We are told that 40 nurses were identified against a set of selection criteria, including age, working experience, sector (public and private) and marital status, in order to capture a range of views and ensure rigour. Of these 40 invited nurses, 22 agreed to be interviewed (in giving this information, the paper refers to Table 3 but this information is provided in Table 4). Beyond saying that the interviews sought to explore two of the eight hypotheses that were not supported by the quantitative findings of the Phase 1 survey, the authors do not provide any further information about the content of the interviews: for example, no topic guide is provided, and we are not told how long the interviews took. It is worth noting that the Phase 1 survey was conducted in October to December 2015, whereas the Phase 2 qualitative in-depth interviews were conducted between December 2016 and February 2017. It is important to consider when the data collection for different components of a mixed methods study are conducted, particularly if they are carried out on the same sample, as it is possible that the nurses' circumstances, perceptions and views may have changed during the intervening period (approximately a year).

We are told that the interviews were conducted by the same investigator, but we are not told of their background or experience. Interviewer background and experience can impact on how questions are asked by the interviewer and how interviewees respond within qualitative interviews. The interviews were audio-taped, transcribed and returned to participants to check for their accuracy. This is often referred to as 'member checking' or 'interviewee transcript review', and is a technique sometimes used within qualitative research to ensure the 'true representation' of the interview data. It is not without its critics, however, as it can sometimes lead to the alteration or removal of relevant data (Hagens et al., 2009), and some researchers argue that once the interview is completed, data should not be revisited by the participant as their story was recorded in response to the interviewer at the time and should therefore stand alone.

Are the details of both the qualitative and quantitative research methods made available to the reader?

Researchers who undertake a mixed methods study face a challenge regarding publication as they need to demonstrate rigour in two different methods within the word count of a standard academic paper (which typically reports only one method). Because of this, researchers sometimes report the two approaches separately in two different papers; however, this is not really 'mixing' the methods, as we described above. In mixed method randomised controlled trials (where there tends to be a lot of quantitative data to report), you often find that most of the data presented is quantitative and only a summary of the qualitative findings provided, but an additional paper reporting the qualitative findings in more detail and depth is also published separately. Where authors present both methods in the same paper, it would therefore not be surprising if some of the detail was not available (although supplementary online material can be provided in most journals). For example, we have observed that Dousin et al. (2021) did not include details about the prior validation of the Phase 1 survey questionnaires, nor how they were distributed and returned, and they did not include detail about the Phase 2 topic guide or questions. This illustrates the difficulty of including all the relevant information for a mixed methods study in a single paper.

Good practice in the reporting of mixed methods research has been described by O'Cathain et al. (2008). O'Cathain et al. (2008) reviewed the reporting of 118 mixed methods studies and found an emphasis on the reporting of the individual components of the studies. They found little evidence of the justification and transparency for the use of mixed methods research; they also found that integration of the results of each method used within a study was limited. Dousin et al. (2021) do provide this justification and hence it is a good example of a mixed methods study.

Who was invited to participate in the study?

The important point to remember is that a mixed methods study comprises separate methods that contribute to one single research study or programme, and participants are recruited according to the needs of each component. There can be a group of participants who take part in both components, or separate unique samples may be used for each component. Dousin et al. (2021) had one sample of nurses who were invited to participate in the Phase 1 survey and, following that, invited a sub-set of these respondents to take part in the Phase 2 qualitative interview study.

How did they analyse the results?

As there are separate research methods within a mixed methods study, data analysis of each needs to be undertaken. Sometimes this is done separately, and then the findings are integrated, or sometimes the findings of the two approaches are analysed together (often using a matrix). Dousin et al.'s (2021) Phase 1 quantitative survey and Phase 2 qualitative interviews were analysed separately. As this is an explanatory, sequential mixed methods study, the quantitative data was analysed first and qualitative data collection and analysis followed, in order to shed light on the results of the quantitative analysis; that is, questions arising from the quantitative survey analysis were explored in the qualitative interviews that followed.

In the quantitative analysis (Phase 1), Dousin et al. (2021) refer the reader back to the hypotheses stated prior to the study. They used the quantitative data from the survey to find out whether the hypothesis could be supported; that is, whether intention to leave was mediated by factors such as job satisfaction, supportive supervision and monetary benefits. Subsequently, in the qualitative data collection (Phase 2), the researchers explored the concepts of monetary benefits and life satisfaction and their effect on nurses' intention to leave in more detail, as the two hypotheses relating to these were not supported by the survey findings – the qualitative analysis therefore focused on this. Whilst the data from each phase was analysed separately in Dousin et al. (2021), the findings arising from Phase 1 informed the design of Phase 2, and the findings of both studies are brought together in the discussion section. The two methods were therefore integrated in the study design.

> The interviewees echoed the empirical evidence that a shortage of nurses in Malaysia is leading to high workloads which eventually decreases nurse well-being and retention in the profession (Atashzaden Shoriden et al., 2012).

How did they present the results?

The data from the Phase 1 quantitative and Phase 2 qualitative study are presented one after the other – in the order that they were collected. The results from the Phase 1 survey are presented and the extent to which they support the hypothesis is discussed. The data suggests that the hypothesis that job satisfaction and supportive supervision affected nurses' intention to leave is supported. However, monetary benefits and life satisfaction did not seem to have an effect on intention to leave. These findings then become the focus of the Phase 2 qualitative data collection and analysis: themes arising from the data are presented, accompanied by supporting quotes to illustrate and provide evidence for them. We have discussed the presentation of data from a survey and a qualitative study in previous chapters (see Chapters 2 and 3 for guidance on this). The results from the survey and qualitative data analysis are merged in the discussion section of the paper – we can therefore observe an integration of the findings.

Was the study ethical?

In a mixed methods study, we need to consider the ethical implications arising from both the quantitative and qualitative methods. Ethical issues associated with survey research were addressed in Chapter 2. Given the high response rate to the questionnaire, it is unclear whether respondents felt some obligation to complete it; there is insufficient information in the paper on the methods used for us to judge this. Ethical issues associated with qualitative interviews were discussed in Chapters 3 and 4. As in the completion of a questionnaire, those participating in interviews should not feel under any obligation to do so. The paper also reports that the study gained relevant ethical approval.

> 2.5 ETHICAL CONSIDERATIONS
>
> The study was approved by RMIT Human Research Ethics Committee and the Ministry of Health, Malaysia Research Ethics Committee.

How confident can we be of the results of the study?

The very high response rate to the Phase 1 survey should give us confidence that the survey's findings represent the views of the population of interest, but the response rate was unusually high which might lead the reader to question whether participants felt obligated to take part and whether this might then have impacted on their responses. However, the nature of their responses (in that they included responses critical of the system) suggests that this was not the case. Further, this mixed methods study reports on the integration of quantitative and qualitative findings which provides additional confidence in the results. These results have special resonance for Malaysia and the specific situation there regarding attrition in the nursing workforce: these factors might be specific only to Malaysia and not apply elsewhere. However, the reader can consider the relevance of the findings to their own particular context.

In summary

This chapter we have identified some of the key features to look for when you are reading a mixed methods study paper. Mixed methods studies should include qualitative and quantitative methods (rather than just multiple qualitative or multiple quantitative methods) – the order of the approaches will depend on the research question or study aims. There are different mixed methods study designs, but a key feature of all mixed methods studies is that the two approaches (quantitative and qualitative) should 'speak' to one another: they should be integrated at some point before the researchers draw any conclusions from the study. This integration can happen at different stages of the research (depending on the aims or research question); for instance, through the study design, sampling or analysis. The conclusion of a mixed methods study should be something that would not have been available without that integration of the two approaches. This paper provided an account of an explanatory mixed methods study; the integration of the findings from the quantitative survey and qualitative interviews provides a comprehensive insight into the intention to leave of nurses in a specific area of Malaysia, developing a deeper understanding than would have been achieved by the use of just one of these methods alone.

BOX 8.1: QUESTIONS TO ASK YOURSELF ABOUT A MIXED METHODS STUDY

When reading a mixed methods paper, always ask:

- Were both qualitative and quantitative approaches used?
- Who took part in each method?
- Were the individual methods used appropriate?
- Were the two approaches integrated at any point?
- Was the study conclusion something that would not have been available without integration?

REFLECTIONS FROM ONE OF THE PAPER'S AUTHORS

We were able to make contact with Pauline Stanton, one of the authors of this paper. Pauline provided very generous feedback on a draft of this chapter, which we have summarised here:

I think that it is a great review of the paper. You have covered all the points. The only thing that I can add is that the Journal of Advanced Nursing is very strict on word count. A mixed methods study means that not only do you have heaps of data but also you have to include details of both methods in the paper. You finally get it down to the word limit and send it off and then the reviewers want changes and often additions so you have to look again at what you can cut out without undermining the integrity of the paper. This paper went through two rounds of revise and resubmits. However, the process was worth it as it is a better paper.

SUGGESTED READING

Moffatt, S., White, M., Mackintosh, J. and Howel, D. (2006) Using quantitative and qualitative data in health services research: What happens when mixed method findings conflict? *BMC Health Services Research*, 6: article no. 28.

Tashakkori, A. and Teddlie, C. (2010) *Sage Handbook of Mixed Methods in Social and Behavioral Research* (2nd edition). Thousand Oaks, CA: Sage Publications.

Teddlie, C. and Yu, F. (2007) Mixed methods sampling: A typology with examples. *Journal of Mixed Methods Research*, 1: 77–100.

9 An integrative review paper

So far in this book, we have been looking at single research studies: empirical studies in which researchers identify a research question and then collect data (most commonly from participants) in order to answer that question. We have seen how research methods can be quantitative (where data is collected and analysed in a numerical format) or qualitative (where data is collected and analysed as a narrative), or use mixed methods, and how the method used depends on the research question. Whichever type of research we are interested in, one study rarely provides enough evidence to be conclusive on a topic or question in its own right – that is, we rarely change practice on the basis of evidence from one research paper. One research study is like one piece of a jigsaw that contributes one piece of evidence to an overall picture. In order to see the whole picture, we need to identify and scrutinise all the relevant papers on a topic, summarise them and make a judgement based on the quality of the resulting evidence that is then available and what it tells us. The formal way of doing this is through a literature review.

In the final two chapters, we will introduce you to two common types of literature review, both of which are established methods for identifying, assessing, summarising and interpreting the results of a body of research to answer a question: a review question as opposed to a research question. Established methods for doing literature reviews should be regarded as research methods in their own right; they have a question which is answered using a systematic method which produces results and leads to discussion and subsequent conclusions.

There are many published methods for doing a literature review; for example, integrative review, systematic review, meta-ethnography and critical interpretative synthesis, to name but a few. These are discussed in detail by Aveyard (2019). The term 'systematic review' has a specific resonance with some researchers and is explored in the next chapter where, for clarity, we refer to this type of review as a 'systematic review with a quantitative meta-analysis'. Some reviews are referred to as systematic reviews because of the explicit method they use to identify, select and synthesise papers, whilst others are not referred to by the term systematic but are none the less undertaken in a systematic way. You may come across other published reviews which have been undertaken in a less thorough or systematic way; these need to be viewed with caution. When you come across any type of review, one thing to check is whether it has a clearly identified method: the researchers should clearly report the method they followed to undertake the review, including which search terms they used, the inclusion and exclusion criteria, which databases they searched, how they assessed the quality of the papers identified (critical appraisal), and how they analysed and synthesised the literature.

In this chapter, we explore an integrative review. An integrative review is used by researchers who need a method that will facilitate the integration of a range of research, and possibly non-research evidence, rather than just one type of evidence such as randomised controlled trials (which we will explore in the next chapter: systematic review with meta-analysis). Whittemore and Knafl (2005) characterise integrative reviews as a type of review with a clearly defined and rigorous method that incorporates both qualitative and quantitative research, in addition to other sources where appropriate. By including, and integrating, both qualitative and quantitative research (experimental and non-experimental studies), these reviews can help answer questions comprehensively by synthesising knowledge to enable evidence-based practice.

The paper we will explore in this chapter is:

Widberg, C., Wiklund, B. and Klarare, A. (2020) Patients' experience of eHealth in palliative care: An integrative review. *BMC Palliative Care*, 19: article no. 158.

Get yourself a copy of the paper, read it through, then work/ read through the rest of the chapter, finding the points we iden- tify in the paper: https://bmcpalliatcare.biomedcentral.com/ track/pdf/10.1186/s12904-020-00667-1.pdf

Scan the QR code to be taken straight to the paper.

What does the abstract and information about the authors tell me?

Just as with papers about empirical studies, the abstract of a review should be a concise account of what was done (and why) and what was found. It should provide enough information to enable you to decide whether to access the paper in full. Abstracts for reviews often follow a similar format to those for empirical research studies (background, method, results and conclusion), but the exact format will depend on the journal it is published in.

We are told that this paper reports on a systematic integrative review of patients' experience of eHealth in palliative care. The method for doing an integrative review does not normally have the prefix 'systematic'; it is likely that the term 'systematic' has been added to emphasise the thorough and systematic approach that has been undertaken, such as searching, identifying and appraising the literature to include in the review – the process the researchers went through. From this, we know to expect a review of the relevant available research that has explored patients' experiences of eHealth when they are receiving palliative care.

ABSTRACT

Background:

With a growing world population, a longer life expectancy, and more deaths due to chronic diseases, the need for palliative care is increasing. Palliative care aims to alleviate suffering and to promote well-being for patients with progressive, incurable disease or injury. E-Health entails using information and communication technology for health care provision. It is unclear how patients experience use of eHealth technology within palliative care.

Methods:

The aim of this study was to describe patients' experiences of eHealth in palliative care. A systematic integrative review was performed using six databases: Cinahl Complete; MEDLINE; PubMed; Psychology and Behavioral Sciences Collection; Nursing and Allied Health; and PsycINFO. Twelve studies met the inclusion criteria of adult patients in palliative care, English language, published 2014–2019: comprising 397 patients. Six studies were from European countries, four from North America, one from South America and one from Oceania. Seven were feasibility or pilot studies.

Results:

The findings are synthesized in the main theme: E-health applications – promoting communication on: patients' and families' terms, and three sub-themes: usability and feasibility of eHealth applications; symptom control and individualized care; and use of eHealth applications increasing the sense of security and patient safety. Patients' experiences were that eHealth promoted individualized care, sense of security, better symptom management and participation in care. Communication was facilitated by the inherent flexibility provided by technology.

Conclusions:

E-Health applications seem promising in promoting equal, individualized care, and may be a tool to endorse accessibility and patient participation in palliative care settings. The indications are that eHealth communication resulted in patients and their families receiving more information, which contributed to their experiences of patient safety and feelings of security. At organizational and societal levels, eHealth may contribute to sustainable development and a more efficient use of resources.

Keywords: eHealth, Literature review, Nursing, Palliative care, Patient

If you look at the keywords at the bottom of the abstract, you will see that this paper has been classified by the authors simply as a literature review. This may be due to limitations in the keywords available for them to select from. Journals ask authors to provide keywords for use by search engines; they are there to ultimately help you find the paper, as we discussed in the introductory chapter. The authors are all registered nurses, working within Swedish university departments, with two of the three employed in palliative care departments.

Is there a clear research question or aim addressed by the review?

A literature review, just like an empirical research study, should have a clear question that guides it: this is sometimes referred to as the review question (rather than the research question). Whilst the title of the paper clearly states the purpose of the review, which is reflected in the stated aim of the study (to describe the evidence regarding patients' experience of eHealth in palliative care), this is not phrased as a question. In an integrative review, the topic or problem can be written as a question or, as in this case, stated as an aim. In this paper, the aim appears at the start of the methods section – sometimes it is set at the end of the background section.

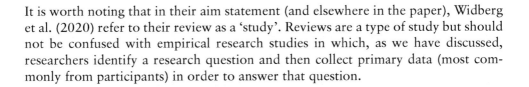

METHODS

The aim of the study was to describe the evidence regarding patients' experiences of eHealth in palliative care.

It is worth noting that in their aim statement (and elsewhere in the paper), Widberg et al. (2020) refer to their review as a 'study'. Reviews are a type of study but should not be confused with empirical research studies in which, as we have discussed, researchers identify a research question and then collect primary data (most commonly from participants) in order to answer that question.

How was the study designed?

The study is described as a systematic integrative review. As with any research study, established reviews have their own methods and should reflect high standards of methodological rigour. The method chosen for doing an integrative review was developed by Whittemore and Knafl (2005), based on the work of Broome (1993), and there have been some suggested developments to the method since then, for example by Christmals and Gross (2017). In the paper we are exploring, Widberg et al. (2020) tell us that they are following the approach to integrative reviews as developed by Whittemore and Knafl (2005); hence we should expect that they are following this established method.

> The study was informed by the outlined steps of Whittmore and Knafl [32], namely problem identification, literature search, data evaluation, data analysis and presentation.

The researchers explain the steps they followed in this method: identification of the problem, which leads to a review question, then the search for literature that will help to answer that review question, the evaluation of that literature, followed by the analysis and presentation of the literature. These steps are explained in detail later in this chapter.

What questions might be asked in an integrative review?

Questions that integrative reviews address are broad ranging. They seek to understand a topic area through systematically assessing, categorising and thematically analysing a diverse body of relevant literature. Integrative reviews have become a popular method of doing a literature review due to the broad approach to the inclusion of evidence. There are methods for doing an exploratory literature review that include only qualitative research: for example, meta-ethnography is one such method. Such an approach would exclude surveys and randomised controlled trials, which are predominantly quantitative in method. Instead, in an integrative review, researchers are asking questions that need to be answered by a broad range of qualitative and quantitative research, sometimes in addition to other forms of evidence such as policy documents or guidelines.

Integrative reviews are not seeking to reduce data in the papers to a single 'yes' or 'no' response in order to answer questions such as 'does this intervention work?'. Neither are researchers seeking to compare, or find associations between, variables – as is often the aim in a systematic review with meta-analysis. Review questions that require comparison or testing for associations across data presented in different research papers (for example, whether a treatment or intervention is effective) are generally answered through a systematic review that uses meta-analysis: a method which is explored in the next chapter.

In addressing their review question (to describe patients' experiences of using eHealth in palliative care), Widberg et al. (2020) sought to provide a broad view of eHealth by investigating the available evidence. It is likely that they therefore anticipated reviewing both qualitative and quantitative research. That is, they expected the review to draw on both surveys of patient experiences and more in-depth interview studies of patient experience, in addition to other evidence as appropriate. Often, researchers have a reasonable understanding of the type of literature that might be available to them (as they will have explored this already in order to justify the need for the review), which informs the method they will use and the searches they then conduct.

How did the researchers identify papers for inclusion in the review?

In conducting an integrative review, there are prescribed processes to follow for identifying relevant research that has focused on a particular area. This requires the detailed searching of discipline-specific academic journal databases in addition to other ways of seeking evidence, such as searching reference lists of identified paper citation tracing, to ensure a comprehensive and strategic search. This is often done with the assistance of an information specialist such as a health-care librarian.

Once the relevant databases have been identified, it is important for researchers doing the review to devise a search strategy to ensure they identify all the relevant research that has been undertaken in the area. An unstructured search will yield many irrelevant hits or can miss key papers. You have probably experienced this yourself when searching using Google or doing a quick search with more specific academic journal databases.

Academic journal databases are constructed by the indexing of research papers using keywords. As we noted above, keywords are identified by authors when they publish a paper and enable a paper to be indexed so that others can retrieve it. You will have seen keywords identified in the research papers referred to in the other chapters in this book. Users of the databases can then identify papers by these keywords, or by asking the database to search for particular words (and synonyms for these words, i.e. words with the same or similar meaning) within the papers – these are often called search terms. Database users can ask the database to look just at the title of papers for these terms, or to look (also) in the abstract, or in the full paper. They can combine these search terms using Boolean logic: that is, using commands such as OR, AND or NOT. The command OR between two search terms will retrieve all the papers that are in the database that include either search term. The command AND will retrieve all the papers that contain both search terms, making it more specific. For example, let's take the key terms *palliative care* and *end of life*. When combined with AND, the search requires that both terms are in or are indexed by the paper (depending on how the search was constructed), which is very specific and might miss out relevant papers that only include one of these terms. If the terms were combined with OR, the search would require just one or other of the terms to be present in any paper and so would identify papers where either palliative care or end of life was included or indexed. The command NOT between two search terms will retrieve all the papers that are in the database that include the first term only when the second term is not present. This can be useful when you are interested in a very specific aspect of a topic, or when you know that when the term you want to search for is used with another term, its meaning is different (and is irrelevant to your search), but using NOT can also exclude some relevant papers and so is used with caution. There are other Boolean operators that can be used, but these three are the most common.

Most databases have a function where search terms can be suggested by the user as free text or by selecting them from a list of predefined headings (known as Medical Subject Headings or MeSH in PubMed), which is a kind of thesaurus of terms, although different databases might use different terminology for these. Using MeSH and synonyms helps to ensure that papers that are not indexed under specific key-words can still be found.

Searching for papers is therefore more complex than we sometimes like to think. So, when you look at a search strategy in a literature review, do consider how the researchers used the AND, OR or NOT or other commands and the impact of these, and think about whether there were any search terms they did not search for, or whether they, in fact, broadened the search too far.

Reviewers also identify inclusion and exclusion criteria. These help to draw up the boundaries for which papers to include within the review and which to exclude – for example, the publication years of papers to be included or the geographical location or language of studies, in addition to specifying the focus and types of studies sought. Inclusion and exclusion criteria clarify the exact remit of the review. Some of these can be included in the search itself but they are also used by the researchers when they consider whether to include the full papers identified from their search, as there can be many false hits (i.e. papers that meet the search terms but which are not actu-ally relevant to the particular topic of interest or review question). Papers retrieved by the database following a search are therefore checked against these inclusion and exclusion criteria to ensure the relevance of the papers included in the review. Although Widberg et al. (2020) were looking for papers about eHealth, they did not define what they meant by eHealth in the methods section of the paper. However, if you look in the background section, they do define it there. They imply eHealth and telemedicine are interchangeable but, in some studies, telehealth could include use of the telephone. They also use different ways of expressing eHealth – sometimes using the alternatives E-Health and e-Health.

E-Health involves the use of information and communication technology (ICT) to provide care, and to transmit health information through the Internet and related technologies [9, 13], irrespective of distance. Other commonly used words are telemedicine and telehealth [14].

Widberg et al. (2020) inform us that they searched CINAHL, PsycINFO and MEDLINE in order to retrieve relevant research papers for their review.

Systematic searches were performed in the following databases: CINAHL Complete, MEDLINE (full text), Nursing and Allied Health database, PsycINFO, Psychology and Behavioral Science Collection, and PubMed using the keywords telemedicine, patients and palliative care, identified as relevant Medical Subject Headings (MeSH). Free text words added to the search were attitude, commu-nication, experience, qualitative, discourse and views (see Table 1) [Figure 9.1].

They identified three core concepts relevant to their question: palliative care, technology and experiences. From these, they used MeSH headings and free text search words (attitude, communication, experience, qualitative, discourse and views) in order to ensure a comprehensive search for relevant papers. Their search strategy is presented in Table 2 of the paper and illustrates how they used the AND and OR commands to conduct their search.

Inclusion and exclusion criteria were also set. The researchers specified that they would search for papers that explored patients' subjective and objective experience of eHealth. Qualitative, quantitative and mixed methods studies were therefore sought. Although the integrative review can incorporate non-research papers, such as policy documents or personal opinion, the researchers in this study did not include any additional forms of evidence. They restricted the search to papers published within the five years prior to the search, due to the rapidly changing nature of the topic under investigation. No geographical limitations were set, but papers had to be published in English or Swedish. The inclusion and exclusion criteria are presented in Table 1 of the paper (Figure 9.1), but a little more detail is in the text; for instance, the words telemedicine, patients and palliative care needed to be in either the title or the abstract.

Table 1 Inclusion and exclusion criteria

Criteria	Inclusion	Exclusion
Types of studies	Qualitative, quantitative, and mixed methods original studies on the phenomenon and with explicit ethical considerations published in peer-reviewed journals	Letters, comments, conference abstracts, editorials, doctoral thesis, or any type of review
Period	January 1, 2014 until March 3, 2019	Before January 1, 2014, and after March 3, 2019
Languages	English and Swedish	All other languages
Type of participants	Patients in a palliative care trajectory regard-less of diagnosis, aged 18 years or older	Patients who are not in a palliative care trajectory, patients younger than 18
Phenomenon of interest	Patients' subjective and objective experiences of eHealth in palliative care	Health care professionals' and families' views on eHealth in palliative care

Figure 9.1   Table 1 from Widberg et al. (2020)

Widberg et al. (2020) reviewed the title and abstract of all papers retrieved by the search against their inclusion and exclusion criteria. This process was undertaken by the first and second authors who then met to resolve any difference of opinion (so they discussed papers they hadn't originally agreed on when they looked at them separately). It is important to record the search for papers and document the decisions made about the papers in the review: the number of records identified, included and excluded, and the reasons for exclusions. One method of documenting this is by using a PRISMA flowchart: see www.prisma-statement.org. PRISMA is the acronym for 'Preferred Reporting Items for Systematic review and Meta Analysis', taken from the work of Moher et al. (2009) in which they described the optimal reporting of systematic reviews with meta-analysis: a method of doing a systematic review which we will discuss in the next chapter. The PRISMA flowchart is a visual way of presenting the decisions made about papers identified from the database search. The PRISMA flowchart is now widely used by many researchers when doing a review, not just those doing a systematic review with meta-analysis. Widberg et al. (2020) used this method to document the search process: their PRISMA flowchart is in Figure 2 of their paper (Figure 9.2).

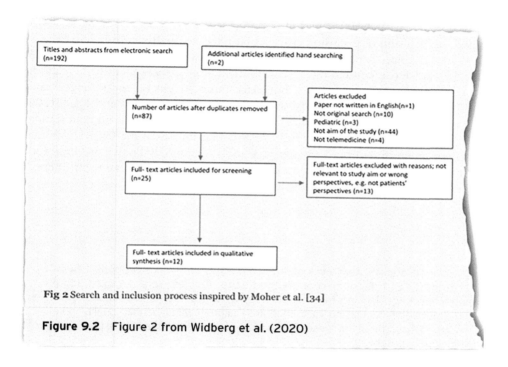

Fig 2 Search and inclusion process inspired by Moher et al. [34]

Figure 9.2   Figure 2 from Widberg et al. (2020)

From Figure 2 of their paper (Figure 9.2), we can see that, from a total number of 194 potentially relevant papers (192 found by the database search and two additional papers found by hand-searching journals), 12 papers were eventually included in the final review. So, there were 12 papers left from that 194 first identified once the duplicates were removed and the inclusion and exclusion criteria were applied. Although a total of 194 papers sounds like a lot, it is actually quite a small number for the identification stage of a review; it is possible that this search might have been too specific and may not have identified some relevant papers. For example, a similar review undertaken by Hancock et al. (2019) identified 3,807 titles and finally included 30 papers.

Did they undertake a critical appraisal of the included papers?

Once the papers for inclusion in a review have been identified, the next stage is to evaluate the quality of the papers: this is sometimes known as critical appraisal.

The purpose of undertaking an appraisal is primarily for the researchers to make a thorough assessment of the quality of the studies conducted; that is, to identify the strengths and weaknesses of each study or paper. At this stage, researchers are not considering the results, but how well the study was conducted and therefore how confident we can be in the conclusions of the papers by examining the strength of the evidence provided by the paper, and therefore how much they can rely on the results in the subsequent analysis. This is important for two reasons. Firstly, some reviewers will set inclusion or exclusion criteria that relate to quality criteria in papers and will therefore reject papers from the review if pre-specified weaknesses are found. Secondly, and more commonly, reviewers include all papers identified, regardless of their strengths and weaknesses, but place more weight on the stronger papers than the weaker papers in the analysis that follows. Whittemore and Knafl (2005) emphasise that critical appraisal of a paper is complex and there is no gold standard for how to do it. Widberg et al. (2020) report that they used the Critical Appraisal Skills Programme suite of critical appraisal tools (commonly known as CASP tools) to evaluate their papers. CASP is just one source of critical appraisal tools; there are many other tools available, covering a range of research designs.

> **DATA EVALUATION**
>
> All included articles were evaluated according to the Critical Appraisal Skills Program (CASP) depending on method used. Articles were not excluded if quality was found lacking, in line with Whittemore and Knafl's recommendations [32]; however, reflection on valid inferences aligned with scientific quality were performed throughout the research process. For details and results of the CASP evaluation, see Table 3.

CASP tools were developed in response to the need to assist practitioners in the evaluation of research and are available at casp-uk.net: there are different CASP tools for different types of research studies, and even for reviews themselves. Widberg et al. (2020) report that they did not use the appraisal to exclude papers from the review: indeed, all of the papers scored highly when scored using relevant CASP tools, and the results of this process are presented in Table 3 of the paper.

How did they analyse the results?

In an integrative review, the analysis of papers is undertaken qualitatively. Whittemore and Knafl (2005) refer to the process of constant comparison, which is an approach used in many qualitative studies (see Chapter 4). Hence, the process of data analysis in an integrative literature review is similar to that undertaken when doing a qualitative analysis of empirical qualitative data, except that, of course, in a literature review, the individual papers are the 'data' that is analysed rather than the empirical data that has been collected from research participants.

In order to analyse the papers in an integrative review, the findings in the results section (and often the insights from the discussion and conclusion) of each included paper are read and re-read. Data that is relevant to the review question is extracted (this is usually called data extraction or data abstraction) and coded. These codes are tentatively assigned to categories and a pattern of meanings generated from across all of the papers begins to emerge to produce themes. As the data analysis progresses, the emergent themes that have been tentatively developed begin to strengthen (as it becomes clear that theme titles reflect their content) or are adapted. As in qualitative research, data analysis is inductive, meaning that researchers are not looking for particular findings, rather the findings emerge: the data in the papers is coded without pre-conceived ideas about their likely content. Researchers sometimes use grids or matrices during this process to help them compare the data or findings across the included studies.

Widberg et al. (2020) refer to taking a qualitative approach to data analysis. Data from the included studies was extracted and pasted into a matrix. This was undertaken by two researchers, initially working independently. Patterns and commonalities were then identified, providing a basis for the development of themes. This is the method advocated by Whittemore and Knafl (2005), as indicated in the extract from Widberg et al. (2020) below. The themes aimed to summarise the findings in a useful way, conveying their underlying meaning.

DATA ANALYSIS

A core in the integrative review, as described by Whittemore and Knafl [32], is the qualitative, iterative nature. As suggested in the data reduction and data display phases, primary data were analyzed and arranged, coded, categorized and summarized in a matrix. This process started with a thorough reading and re-reading of the included articles, performed independently by two persons. Each person extracted data relevant to the aim and pasted it into a matrix, initially assessing each article by itself, and later discussing the findings. In the data comparison phase, patterns and commonalities were noted, grouped together and contrasted in line with shifting perspectives to allow critical analysis of data. A thorough and impartial interpretation of data, promotes innovative synthesis of evidence [32], one goal of the data analysis step. This process of shifting perspectives and noting commonalities and patterns resulted in the creation of a main theme: E-health applications – promoting communication on patients' and families' terms, and three sub-themes. The themes were created based on groupings of: findings, aiming to summarize the synthesis, and putting it into words that conveyed the underlying meaning, to present in a useful way to a wider audience [35].

How did they present the results?

Widberg et al. (2020) initially summarise the 12 papers, stating which countries they come from, and key characteristics (for example, age and diagnoses) of participants in the included papers (397 in total), the context where the care took place (for example, a hospice or a hospital ward) and the types of eHealth investigated. They present a summary of the 12 included papers in Table 4 of the paper (note that they describe this as a 'matrix', but this should not be confused with the analytic matrix referred to in the methods). This provides the reader with a useful overview, or summary, of the individual research papers that are included in the review. However, the purpose of an integrative review is to present an analysis and synthesis of the findings of the relevant papers in order to answer the review question, rather than to just present the individual papers to the reader. The presentation of the papers in Table 4 is therefore for the interest of the reader as background and is a prelude to the results of the combined analysis of the papers. We are also given a breakdown of the numbers of qualitative, quantitative and mixed methods studies and their country of origin. The actual findings of the analysis of papers are presented in the rich thematic narrative which follows.

The findings are presented in the form of themes that had been identified according to the method described in the previous section. Unusually, there is a single main theme ('eHealth applications – promoting communication on patients' and families' terms') and three sub-themes relating to the useability of eHealth, the use of eHealth for symptom control, and the safety and security of eHealth. Each sub-theme is supported by relevant data which has been extracted from each of the papers. The data within each sub-theme is compared to each other so that each sub-theme represents the meaning derived from the relevant papers, and clear reference is given to the papers that have contributed to each sub-theme.

Was the study ethical?

When undertaking a literature review, ethical issues are less extensive than when undertaking an empirical study; researchers are not collecting data from potentially vulnerable people where there is potential for harm. Instead, they are bringing together and reviewing the work of others, using studies which have already been published. Publication of the individual papers included in the review usually requires that those individual studies have been reviewed and approved by an ethical committee, but this should not be assumed. Also, it is still possible to identify ethical issues within a literature review. The question of how researchers should act if they encounter a study that does not appear to have been undertaken in an ethical manner is an important one and consideration given as to whether it should be included in the review or removed. It can be argued that if harm has already been done by the undertaking of the study, there is nothing further to be gained by excluding it from the review (and it might be unethical to exclude it). Alternatively, it might be argued that further harm may be done to the participants by its inclusion. This needs to be judged on a case-by-case basis; it remains a judgement call and at the discretion of the reviewers.

The other question is the fair representation of the paper within the review when the paper, or data within the paper, is analysed. Those undertaking a literature review are obliged to represent the work of others accurately and fairly, without emphasising certain aspects of the data more than others. Of course, the purpose of a review is to remove the requirement for a reader to read every included paper, and so there remains an element of trust that papers have been appropriately represented.

Unusually for a review, Widberg et al. (2020) included 'explicitly stated ethical considerations' as an inclusion criterion for their review, but in practice we don't know how they assessed this.

ETHICS APPROVAL AND CONSENT TO PARTICIPATE

Not relevant for an integrative review; however, ethical considerations in the studies were included in the review process.

How confident can we be of the findings?

Just as with an empirical research paper, it is important that the discussion section of a review paper is not simply a repeat of the results. Ideally, the discussion in a literature review should not exclusively refer back to the included papers but should refer to other parallel sources that help to explain what the results might mean. It should also present the strengths and limitations of the review process itself. For example, in an integrative review, the results are dependent on the quality of the searching – here it is worth considering whether the lack of a definition for eHealth might have limited the results obtained. In acknowledging the potential limitations of the review, Widberg et al. (2020) refer to the broader concepts of accessing health care and relate their findings to an identified model, thus broadening the discussion beyond the findings of their analysis, contributing to wider generalisable concepts.

There are a number of limitations to consider in this study. A plethora of different terms are used within the area of eHealth, and it is possible that some terms were missed in our search strategies.

In summary

In this chapter we have identified some of the key features to look for when you are reading an integrative review. Review papers identify, assess, summarise and synthesise the results of a body of research to answer a question: a review question as opposed to a research question. Integrative reviews bring together a range of research evidence, and possibly non-research evidence, rather than just one type (such as RCTs). An analysis of papers is undertaken qualitatively, and the findings are usually reported as a narrative. How the included papers are found and assessed is crucial to the outcome of the review. In this review paper, Widberg et al. (2020) report on a systematic integrative review of patients' experience of eHealth in palliative care. It presents a rich thematic narrative located in the broader concepts of accessing health care.

BOX 9.1: QUESTIONS TO ASK YOURSELF ABOUT AN INTEGRATIVE REVIEW

When reading an integrative review, always ask:

- Is there a clear review question?
- Was there a clear and appropriate search strategy (databases, search terms, inclusion and exclusion criteria)?
- Is the result of the search process reported (e.g. using a PRISMA flow diagram)?
- Did the authors conduct critical appraisal and how did they use the findings of that appraisal?
- How did they assess and synthesise the findings of the included papers?

REFLECTIONS FROM ONE OF THE PAPER'S AUTHORS

We were able to make contact with Anna Klarare, one of the authors of this paper. Anna provided very generous feedback on a draft of this chapter, with particular reference to the use of the CASP appraisal tools, which we have summarised here:

We found that CASP provided structure but did not really pinpoint methodological weaknesses. It is likely that doing more in-depth analysis with another tool, and highlighting this in the method, would be helpful.

SUGGESTED READING

Flemming, K. and Noyes, J. (2021) What is qualitative evidence synthesis? Where are we at? *International Journal of Qualitative Methods*. [online]

Noyes, J., Booth, A., Moore, G., Flemming, K., Tunçalp, Ö. and Shakibazadeh, E. (2019) Synthesising quantitative and qualitative evidence to inform guidelines on complex interventions: Clarifying the purposes, designs and outlining some methods. *BMJ Global Health*, 4 (Suppl. 1): article no. e000893. https://doi.org/10.1136/bmjgh-2018-000893

Whittemore, R. and Knafl, K. (2005) The integrative review; updated methodology. *International Journal of Nursing Studies*, 52(5): 546–53.

10 A systematic review with meta-analysis paper

In the previous chapter, we looked at an example of a literature review in which relevant papers on a topic were collected and reviewed together to synthesise the available evidence to answer a review question. This process enables the reader to have an understanding of the body of research on the focused topic or question, rather than just one piece of research in isolation; the analogy that one piece of research can be regarded as just one piece of a jigsaw is useful here. The example we looked at was an integrative review, in which different types of evidence, including research and non-research evidence such as policy and guidelines, can be incorporated. Integrative reviews are a popular form of review due to their inclusive nature and the diverse range of evidence they can include. Due to the diverse range of evidence in the review, the analysis and reporting of papers are generally undertaken as a narrative: usually through some sort of thematic analysis of the findings of the included papers.

In this chapter, we will be looking at a different type of review: a systematic review that uses meta-analysis. This type of review has a very specific purpose: its aim is to determine the effectiveness of a treatment or an intervention by combining and re-analysing together the results of several quantitative studies – most often randomised controlled trials. This process produces a summary statistic relating to all the studies combined, providing an overall overview of the effectiveness of the intervention. This is often referred to as a meta-analysis. Researchers also provide a narrative summary to supplement this overall statistical result, but the intention of a meta-analysis is to provide a precise statistical re-analysis of the combined quantitative results of the existing studies so that the effectiveness from the results of different studies (which are the equivalent of a larger sample) can be determined.

The systematic review with meta-analysis is the 'original' systematic review design. It is argued to be one of the most influential factors on the development of methods for the other types of literature review which then followed, such as the integrative review (Aveyard et al., 2021). The systematic review with meta-analysis was developed by the work of the Cochrane Collaboration, founded by Professor Archie Cochrane, who argued convincingly that the lack of good evidence upon which many commonly used medical treatments and interventions were based was a concern (Cochrane, 1972). This challenge resulted in the foundation of the Cochrane Collaboration (www.cochrane.org/about-us) which uses this approach to gather and synthesise the best evidence from research to help make informed choices about treatments. It produces high-quality, relevant, up-to-date systematic reviews and other synthesised research evidence to inform health decision making. There are over 7,500 published Cochrane Systematic Reviews, most of which are systematic reviews with a meta-analysis.

The type of study included in a systematic review with meta-analysis is most often the randomised controlled trial (RCT) – a research design we discussed in Chapter 6. The RCT is the only type of study design that can establish causation: in other words, whether a treatment or an intervention influences a pre-determined outcome – so, whether it works or not. RCTs do this by allocating participants into groups who receive different treatments or interventions, then following them up to measure outcomes. A systematic review with meta-analysis incorporates all the studies that have compared the same or similar intervention or treatment in order to answer a clinical question related to that intervention. It provides an analysis of a whole body of evidence rather than just one RCT. Most Cochrane Collaboration systematic reviews with meta-analysis therefore bring together all the RCTs that have been undertaken up to that point in time that might answer a specific clinical question relating to a particular intervention or treatment.

As discussed in Chapter 9, it is not uncommon to find that literature reviews are published and indexed using different labels (Aveyard and Bradbury-Jones, 2019), and the systematic review with meta-analysis is no exception to this. For example, you might find that these papers are referred to as 'a systematic review' or 'a meta-analysis' or 'a Cochrane systematic review'. As we discussed in the previous chapter, the important point is to be able to recognise the type of review from the method described in the paper and to know the key features to look out for and appraise in it. In this chapter, we will therefore discuss the method used by those undertaking a systematic review with meta-analysis. The paper we are referring to in this chapter is:

Smigorowsky, M. J., Sebastianski, M., Sean McMurtry, M., Tsuyuki, R. T. and Norris, C. M. (2020) Outcomes of nurse practitioner-led care in patients with cardiovascular disease: A systematic review and meta-analysis. *Journal of Advanced Nursing*, 76(1): 81–95.

Get yourself a copy of the paper, read it through, then work/read through the rest of the chapter, finding the points we identify in the paper: https://onlinelibrary.wiley.com/doi/pdf/10.1111/jan.14229

Scan the QR code to be taken straight to the paper.

What does the abstract and information about the authors tell me?

Just as with empirical papers, the abstract of a review should be a concise summary of why the review was done, what was done, what was found and what it means: it should provide enough information to enable you to decide whether to access the paper in full. Smigorowsky et al.'s (2020) abstract informs us of an existing gap in knowledge about the effectiveness of nurse-led care in patients with cardiovascular disease, as no previous systematic reviews on this issue could be identified. Indeed, it also hints at the paucity of studies in the area as we are told that only five studies met the review's inclusion criteria, suggesting that the results of the review might be limited and, indeed, this is what was concluded.

ABSTRACT

Aim:

To assess randomized controlled trials evaluating the impact of nurse practitioner-led cardiovascular care.

Background:

Systematic review of nurse practitioner-led care in patients with cardiovascular disease has not been completed.

Design:

Systematic review and meta-analysis.

Data sources:

The Cochrane Central Register of Controlled Trials (CENTRAL), Medline, Embase, CINAHL, Web of Science, Scopus and ProQuest were systematically searched for studies published between January 2007–June 2017.

Review methods:

Cochrane methodology was used for risk of bias, data extraction and meta-analysis. The quality of evidence was assessed using Grading of Recommendations Assessment, Development and Evaluation approach.

Results:

Out of 605 articles, five articles met the inclusion criteria. There was no statistical difference between nurse practitioner-led care and usual care for 30-day readmissions, health-related quality of life and length of stay. A 12% reduction in Framingham risk score was identified.

Conclusion:

There are a few randomized control trials assessing nurse practitioner-led cardiovascular care.

Impact:

Low to moderate quality evidence was identified with no statistically significant associated outcomes of care. Nurse practitioner roles need to be supported to conduct and publish high-quality research.

Keywords: Cardiovascular care, Clinical intervention, Meta-analysis, Nurse, Nurse practitioner, Outcomes of care, Randomized control trial, Systematic review

The abstract (and the paper's title) clearly states that this is a systematic review and meta-analysis. It tells us which databases were searched, and for what time period. It also gives an overview of how the papers were assessed for their quality, how the data was extracted from the papers and how it was synthesised (combined). It summarises the results and provides a concluding statement, in addition to a statement on impact: what the findings mean for clinical practice and research.

Information about the authors tells us that they are academics and clinicians from a range of professions (including nursing), from clinical and university departments in Alberta, Canada. For a review, this does not mean that the empirical studies included in the review were only undertaken in Canada, it is simply that the team who conducted the review was located there. Depending on their remit, systematic reviews often bring together international studies. Clearly, there are some topics that lend themselves to an international remit and some that do not (e.g. those that are specific to a particular type of health system, cultural or country-specific question do not usually lend themselves to an international remit). It is clear from information presented later in the review that an international focus was intended for it.

Is there a clear research question or aim addressed by the review?

A literature review, just like an empirical research study, will usually have a clear question that guides the review: this is sometimes referred to as the review question or the research question or, alternatively, the focus of the review might be expressed as an aim. Smigorowsky et al.'s (2020) aim was to assess the evidence on nurse practitioner-led cardiovascular care and the associated outcomes of care; they wanted to assess the effectiveness of this type of care by conducting a systematic review and meta-analysis. They also state this as a research (review) question:

2.1 AIM

This systematic review and meta-analysis aimed to appraise the existing evidence related to the effectiveness of cardiovascular nurse practitioner-led care (as a model of care) on the outcomes of care for adult patients. The research question is: what are the outcomes of care associated with cardiovascular nurse practitioner-led care?

The rationale behind the review question is clearly articulated in the introduction and background sections of the paper. Health care systems around the world are facing increasing patient demand due to demographic changes and need to identify the most cost-effective ways of delivering care. As the role of the nurse develops (including the development of advanced roles such as nurse practitioners), identifying optimal ways in which nurses can provide care is important. One way to do this is to evaluate nurse practitioner-led clinics and to compare patient outcomes against more traditional medically led clinics. If patient (and cost) outcomes are similar, or better, we can deduce that nurse practitioner-led clinics provide an equivalent (cost-effective) level of patient care. Therefore, if we are interested in finding out about outcomes from nurse practitioner-led clinics, we need to review all studies that have compared outcomes from nurse practitioner-led clinics and from traditional clinics and combine these in a meta-analysis. Before embarking on this, the background section of the paper also tells us about other reviews that have been conducted which are aligned to the review question, but which do not completely answer it – this justifies and sets the scene for the review.

How was the study designed?

The study is described as a systematic review and meta-analysis of RCTs. This means that the authors were seeking to combine the quantitative results of all RCTs that have evaluated patient outcomes from this type of nurse practitioner-led clinic. The term meta-analysis indicates that the quantitative data from across the included studies were combined and analysed together in order to produce one summary statistic that captures the combined findings of all the studies.

2.2 DESIGN

This research was conducted by completing a SR of RCTs reporting NPs providing care in CV patient care settings and examining the impact of clinical outcomes of care associated with NP-led care using the guidelines of the Cochrane Collaboration (Higgins et al., 2019) and reported using Preferred Reporting Items for Systematic Reviews and Meta-Analyses (PRISMA) statement (Moher et al., 2015).

In Smigorowsky et al. (2020), the authors refer to the Cochrane handbook for systematic reviews as the foundation for their work (Higgins et al., 2019). The handbook provides detailed guidance for those doing this very specific type of literature review. Despite the specific nature of the review, the design of a systematic review with meta-analysis has many similarities to the integrative review we discussed in Chapter 9. In both types of review, the researchers have a review question or aim; they then undertake a systematic search, appraise the identified papers and extract the relevant data. It is at the point of analysis of the combined findings of the papers that the method for doing a systematic review with meta-analysis differs from other reviews. The approach to analysis in a systematic review with meta-analysis is statistical; the meta-analysis is the statistical procedure that is undertaken to analyse the combined quantitative findings of all of the studies (or papers) included in the review. The purpose is to determine the overall effectiveness of a treatment or an intervention (in this case, a type of nurse practitioner-led care) and this can be done from looking at the results from across all of the papers, then pooling and analysing them. The purpose is to produce an overall summary statistic from the included papers.

Many authors of systematic reviews with a meta-analysis publish a review protocol ahead of conducting the review. These can be published in a repository such as PROSPERO (www.crd.york.ac.uk) which is one of several international databases of review protocols. The reason for this is to ensure that the academic community is aware of systematic reviews that are in progress (to avoid duplication) and to reduce reporting bias (when findings are selectively reported – and some suppressed – depending on the results) as it provides a permanent record of what was initially planned. Other types of review (such as integrative reviews) can also be registered on these databases, but many journals state this as a requirement for publication of a systematic review with meta-analysis in particular. In this study, the protocol was not published in advance. Furthermore, when writing up a systematic review, there are reporting guidelines that researchers can use to guide their writing up of the study. Examples of reporting guidelines can be found on the EQUATOR website (www.equator-network.org).

What questions might be asked in a systematic review with meta-analysis?

A systematic review with meta-analysis seeks to address questions about the effectiveness, or cost-effectiveness, of a treatment or an intervention, not just from one study but from all relevant and appropriately designed and conducted studies that have been undertaken. Smigorowsky et al.'s (2020) review question was, 'What are the outcomes of care associated with cardiovascular nurse practitioner-led care?' This is an appropriate question for a systematic review with meta-analysis. A similar question will have been asked in the individual RCTs that were combined in the systematic review with meta-analysis.

How did the researchers identify papers for inclusion in the review?

The search strategy for a systematic review with meta-analysis reflects that of other reviews whose aim is to undertake a comprehensive search for papers that are relevant to the review question. It is important to note that the search strategy for a systematic review with meta-analysis is pre-specified at the planning stage of the study and is often published in a protocol, as described above. This often follows an initial scoping of the published literature to explore the likely nature and volume of research available. This can help the researchers decide on aspects of the search strategy (e.g. databases and search terms to use), the parameters for the review (e.g. timeframes to search) and its inclusion and exclusion criteria.

> All published and unpublished RCTs related to CV NP-led care and associated outcomes of care between January 2007 and July 2017 (years) were identified in the following databases: CINAHL, EMBASE, Medline, ProQuest Dissertations & Thesis Global, the Cochrane Central Register of Controlled Trials (CENTRAL), Scopus and Web of Science Core Collection. We consulted with a librarian familiar with nursing and medical research when we developed and conducted the search.

In Chapter 9, we discussed the rationale for undertaking a comprehensive search and how this is undertaken. Smigorowsky et al. (2020) list the databases they searched and inform us of additional search strategies (e.g. searching the reference lists of included papers for relevant additional papers also meeting the inclusion criteria but which were not identified in the main database search). They developed and undertook the pre-specified search with the assistance of a subject academic librarian. Inclusion criteria focused on published or unpublished RCTs in which nurse practitioner-led care was compared with care delivered by another health care provider. Reference to unpublished RCTs probably means data from PhD theses, given that the authors searched a database that has access to dissertations and theses. Patient outcomes associated with nurse practitioner-led care included change in symptoms or quality indicators such as waiting times, length of stay or patient satisfaction. They combined relevant MeSH terms (Medical Subject Headings – see Chapter 9) and keywords. The search was limited to those published in English and within the 10 years prior to the search, on the basis that the provision of care has substantially changed since this period and is continuing to do so. Justifying the decisions made in the design of the review is important – we need to know why the criteria were decided on as they will influence (a) what papers are found and included (or excluded), (b) what the review's findings are, and (c) its conclusion.

The protocol for those doing a systematic review with meta-analysis often requires that two people are involved in all the stages; for example, the searching, the selection of papers and the data extraction. Where the researchers do not agree on the inclusion or relevance of the studies, this is usually resolved by discussion or consultation of a third reviewer. This increases the rigour of the study. The role of the authors in the process of searching and reviewing the papers, and the extent of agreement between the research team about the inclusion of papers in the review, are not reported in this paper; however, Smigorowsky et al. (2020) do report that data extraction was conducted by two authors independently and disagreements dealt with by consensus.

2.6 DATA ABSTRACTION

Study data were extracted by two authors independently and disagreements were dealt with by consensus.

As discussed in Chapter 9, the process of the selection of papers is often recorded in a PRISMA flow diagram: http://prisma-statement.org/prismastatement/flowdiagram.aspx. This documents how many papers were initially identified, how many abstracts were screened and how many full-text papers were obtained and checked in detail against the inclusion criteria. Although this flow diagram does not allow the reader to scrutinise the decisions made, it does report the number and source of records identified, the number included and excluded, and (sometimes) the reasons for exclusions. Smigorowsky et al. (2020) provide a PRISMA flow diagram in Figure 1 of their paper (Figure 10.1).

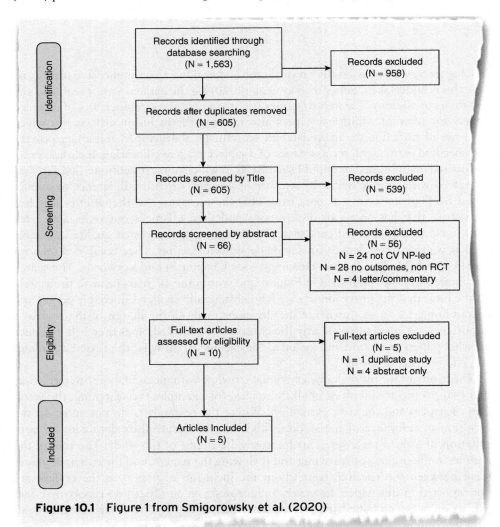

Figure 10.1 Figure 1 from Smigorowsky et al. (2020)

Did they undertake an appraisal of the included papers?

The quality of the papers that are included in a review is an important consideration for any type of review. If all of the included papers are high quality, greater confidence can be placed in the results of the review. We might be less confident in the results of a review that included poorer-quality papers. In Chapter 9, we discussed assessing the quality of a range of papers that might be included in an integrative review and the potential need to use a range of critical appraisal tools to match the designs of the included papers. For a systematic review with meta-analysis, which usually contains only RCTs, the included studies are more similar in design and so can often be assessed using a single tool. Smigorowsky et al. (2020) used the Cochrane Risk of Bias Tool (Higgins et al., 2019) which allows the assessor to identify studies with a low to high risk of bias. Risk of bias is primarily concerned with how objective the methods used were in relation to the randomisation procedure (for example, truly random using a computer-generated randomisation rather than, for example, randomising by the day of the week patients attended a clinic), how participants were allocated (for example, using sealed opaque envelopes to reveal their allocation rather than checking an open list), blinding (for example, knowing who knew which treatment the participant received – including the patient, the treatment team and those analysing the results), how complete the dataset was (for example, how much data was missing and whether it was similar in both arms of the study) and, finally, whether everything was reported. Subgroup analysis can sometimes be conducted with studies with a low risk of bias in order to see how much difference the risk of bias makes to the outcome of the analysis. Of the five studies Smigorowsky et al. (2020) included, two were low risk of bias, two were moderate and one was high risk of bias: they report this in the text and illustrate it in Figures 2 and 3 of the paper. The researchers also refer back to the quality of evidence in the strengths and limitations section.

Smigorowsky et al. (2020) also used GRADE (Grading of Recommendations, Assessment, Development and Evaluations; Guyatt et al., 2011) which is an estimate of how certain you can be about the results of the review. It involves looking at a range of factors including risk of bias, imprecision, inconsistency, indirectness and publication bias, as well as three other criteria: magnitude of effect, dose response and confounding. You don't need to understand exactly what this means but it is useful to check to see if GRADE was used and to look at the level of certainty the reviewers have given for their findings as a result. You might like to take a look at: https://bestpractice.bmj.com/info/toolkit/learn-ebm/what-is-grade.

In addition to appraising the included studies, the relevant data from the studies was extracted from the papers and charted on a data abstraction or data extraction chart. This is a chart which is devised by the researchers to enable them to record and summarise the relevant data from all of the included studies in one place; this then facilitates analysis. Two reviewers also conducted this stage.

How did they analyse the results?

In this type of review, the results within the individual studies are combined and analysed in a statistical test known as a meta-analysis. A meta-analysis relates to

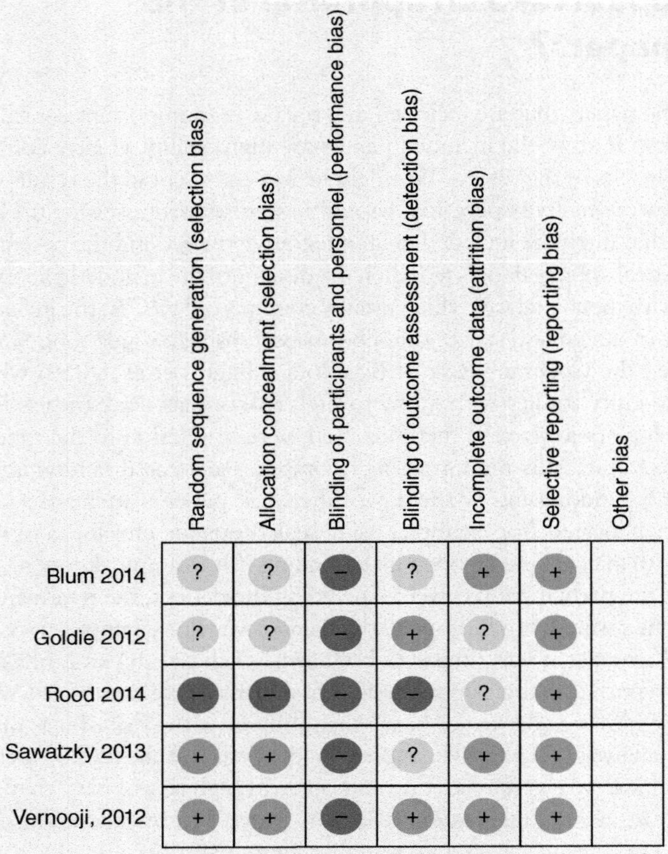

	Random sequence generation (selection bias)	Allocation concealment (selection bias)	Blinding of participants and personnel (performance bias)	Blinding of outcome assessment (detection bias)	Incomplete outcome data (attrition bias)	Selective reporting (reporting bias)	Other bias
Blum 2014	?	?	−	?	+	+	
Goldie 2012	?	?	−	+	?	+	
Rood 2014	−	−	−	−	?	+	
Sawatzky 2013	+	+	−	?	+	+	
Vernooji, 2012	+	+	−	+	+	+	

Figure 10.2 Figure 3 from Smigorowsky et al. (2020)

combining findings on an outcome from similar studies to get an overall outcome, based on analysis of the pooled results of the included studies. This means that effect sizes of individual studies – that is, differences between the comparison groups in a RCT – are combined to form a summary statistic to show the effect size across all of the included studies. Typical effect sizes utilised are measured using terms such as risk ratio, relative risk and odds ratio. Meta-analysis is only an appropriate form of analysis in a systematic review if the papers adopt a similar method and have measured similar outcomes; that is, only studies that are similar enough in relation to key features, such as outcome measures used or populations studied, can be compared. This is sometimes referred to as homogeneity; researchers will usually state that the findings of studies are too different from one another could not be combined.

Smigorowsky et al. (2020) undertook a meta-analysis for four of the five outcomes that their review identified (one outcome – vascular risk reduction – was only reported in one RCT so results relating to it could not be pooled with those from any other RCTs). The four outcomes that underwent meta-analysis were the effects of nurse practitioner-led clinics on: (1) 30-day readmission, (2) length of stay, and (3) physical and (4) mental health of the patient. To do this, Smigorowsky et al. (2020) used specialist review software to conduct the analysis called RevMan, which was developed by the Cochrane Collaboration (www. Cochrane.org).

How did they present the results?

As is standard practice, Smigorowsky et al. (2020) started by describing, or characterising, the five RCTs which they included in their review. Five is a relatively small number for a systematic review with meta-analysis. Two RCTs were from Canada, two from the USA and one from The Netherlands. The authors provide a narrative or description of the RCTs' characteristics as a group and summarise key features of each RCT in a table (Table 1 of the paper) so that the reader has an overview and can assess the individual studies that are included in the analysis.

The results of the meta-analysis are reported in the text but also presented in four figures (Figures 4, 5, 6 and 7 of the paper) – one for each outcome. These figures are known as forest plots and are the standard way to visually present the results of meta-analyses. Forest plots can summarise almost all the essential information from a meta-analysis. They might seem complex at first glance and difficult to understand; however, once you understand what the different parts of the plot represent, the concepts involved are relatively simple.

When you look at a forest plot, all the individual studies are listed on the left-hand side. The result of each study (in relation to the particular outcome of interest) is represented by the solid square in the middle of the horizontal line. The horizontal line represents the confidence intervals for each study. The confidence intervals can be taken to represent the level of certainty about the results of the study; that is, shorter confidence intervals usually indicate that we can be more confident about the results of the study. A line of 'no effect' runs vertically down the middle of the chart. Any study where the confidence intervals cross this line indicates that there is no evidence of a difference between the two groups in the study, so it is a non-significant result. The weight of each study is presented as a percentage, which reflects how strongly each study contributes to the overall average effect estimate. Larger studies tend to have greater weight, as you can imagine, as their findings are less likely to be based on chance. More precise studies, those with narrower confidence intervals, contribute more weight to the overall summary statistic. The diamond represents the average of all studies' results and can be considered to be the overall 'result'.

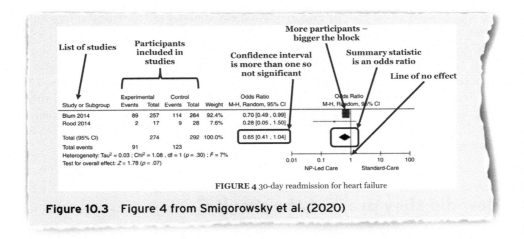

FIGURE 4 30-day readmission for heart failure

Figure 10.3   Figure 4 from Smigorowsky et al. (2020)

In each of Smigorowsky et al. (2020)'s meta-analyses, the summary statistic, represented by the diamond, sits across the line of no effect, indicating that there are no significant differences in patient outcomes from care in a nurse practitioner-led clinic compared to a traditional physician-led one. That is, care was neither significantly better nor worse when the patient attended the nurse practitioner-led clinic. Given the review question, this can be regarded as a good outcome for this review: it suggests that nurse practitioner-led clinics were just as good as physician-led ones (although some caution is needed due to the quality and quantity of the data).

Was the study ethical?

As noted in Chapter 9, ethical issues when undertaking a literature review are less extensive than when undertaking an empirical study but remain important to consider. Our discussion on this in Chapter 9, in relation to integrative reviews, is equally relevant to systematic reviews with meta-analysis. When undertaking meta-analysis, the identification and inclusion of all ethical studies that meet the inclusion criteria are especially important as missing and/or fraudulent studies will create an incomplete picture (Urquhart et al., 2017).

How confident can we be of the results of the systematic review and meta-analysis?

In their discussion, Smigorowsky et al. (2020) explain how the need to evaluate the effectiveness of nurse practitioner-led clinics is a priority given the rising demands of health care, and hence emphasise the importance of the need for evidence of this type.

The researchers concluded that there was a lack of high-quality data: whilst they can tentatively say that the outcomes for patients who attend nurse practitioner-led clinics are equal to those who attend physician-led clinics, they cannot be entirely sure as the quality and quantity of the data available, and therefore included, could have been better. It is also worth noting that nurse practitioner-led care is associated with many positive patient outcomes which were not formally evaluated in the review.

In summary

In this chapter we have identified some of the key features to look for when you are reading a systematic review with meta-analysis. This type of review aims to determine the effectiveness of a treatment or an intervention by combining and re-analysing together the results of several quantitative studies – most often randomised controlled trials – using meta-analysis. The findings are usually reported in tables and figures with a supporting narrative. As with all types of review, how the included papers are found and assessed is crucial to the outcome of the review. In this review, Smigorowsky et al. (2020) assessed the effectiveness of nurse practitioner-led cardiovascular care and the associated outcomes of care compared to physician-led clinics: outcomes for patients who attended nurse practitioner-led clinics were found to be at least equal to those who attend physician-led clinics based on the available data.

BOX 10.1: QUESTIONS TO ASK YOURSELF ABOUT A SYSTEMATIC REVIEW STUDY

When reading a systematic review paper, always ask:

- Is there a clear review question?
- Was there a clear and appropriate search strategy (databases, search terms, inclusion and exclusion criteria)?
- Is the result of the search process reported (e.g. using a PRISMA flow diagram)?
- Did they conduct a critical appraisal and how did they use the findings of that appraisal?
- How did they synthesise the findings of the included papers?

REFLECTIONS FROM ONE OF THE PAPER'S AUTHORS

We were able to make contact with Marcie Smigorowsky, the lead author of this paper. Marcie provided very generous feedback on a draft of this chapter, which we have summarised here:

(Continued)

Marcie shared that this review was preceded by a scoping review and the systematic review informed their subsequent empirical work: a randomised controlled trial of nurse practitioner-led care compared to cardiologist care. From this, you can see that Marcie has built a programme of research around this topic – she described this as each piece of research informing the next level of research, and this is often what happens following a systematic review.

Marcie wanted to clarify the importance of the terms used in the review; in particular, she wanted us to emphasise the distinction between the term nurse-led and nurse practitioner-led as the two terms have different meanings and this is an important distinction in understanding the work. She described nurse practitioner roles as one of the roles typically described as advanced practice nursing (the other is the clinical nurse specialist). In nurse-led, as opposed to nurse practitioner-led, clinics, the nurses are not independent – they function in some association with a physician or multidisciplinary team, sometimes using protocols or algorithms which they must follow, and so are not as independent in their clinical decision making (i.e. diagnosing or prescribing medications or treatments) as nurse practitioners are. Marcie said that although the review showed no difference in care, there were still learnings for future research.

SUGGESTED READING

Higgins, J. P. T., Thomas, J., Chandler, J., Cumpston, M., Li, T., Page, M. J. and Welch, V. A. (eds) (2022) *Cochrane Handbook for Systematic Reviews of Interventions*, version 6.3 (updated February 2022). Available from www.training.cochrane.org/handbook

11 In summary

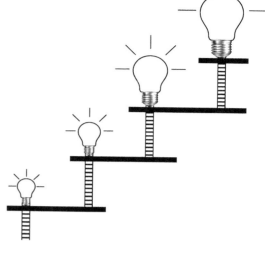

In this book, we have discussed a range of research papers that report on a range of research approaches and designs, identifying key points to look out for in each. There are many methods for doing research and the appropriate method depends on the question being addressed; no method is better or worse than any other – the important consideration is that the method helps answer the research question. If you want to explore experience in an in-depth way, a qualitative approach is likely to facilitate this more than a quantitative one. A survey is useful when shorter answers will help you answer the question. The well-known 'hierarchy of evidence', which we discussed in Chapter 1, only applies to questions about effectiveness. There are other hierarchies for other types of research questions. The most important point to remember is that the first consideration to make about any paper you read is whether the research method reflects the question.

Quantitative research designs are fairly standard and have a defined and consistent approach. Many qualitative research designs are still developing and might be used more flexibly according to the needs of a particular study; hence, it is not unusual to read something like 'this study was informed by grounded theory' and to find that it does not fully adhere to the full principles of that design. You will increasingly come across mixed methods research as we acknowledge that many clinically relevant questions cannot be fully answered by one single method, and benefit from combining and integrating approaches in one study or across a programme of research. At other times, you might want to read a review which summarises all research papers that have addressed a particular issue – the type of review will depend on the review question.

The broad questions we have asked of the papers in each chapter – the sub-headings (summarised in Box 11.1) – can be asked of other research you might come across. They can act as a checklist of questions for your future reading. There are lots of other research designs beyond those covered in this book, but the questions we have posed can be applied to most.

BOX 11.1: KEY QUESTIONS YOU COULD ASK OF EVERY PAPER

- What does the abstract and information about the authors tell me?
- Is there a clear research question or aim addressed by the research?
- How was the study designed?
- What data was collected and how?
- How did the authors analyse the results?

As we saw in the previous two chapters, there are more formal checklists that can help us ask appropriate questions of research papers in order to assess the strengths and weaknesses of a paper. These are often referred to as critical appraisal tools. Some tools are specific to certain research methods, whilst others are generic and apply to the most common designs. Two well-known and well-established instruments are the CASP suite of tools and the Joanna Briggs set of tools:

https://casp-uk.net/casp-tools-checklists

https://jbi.global/critical-appraisal-tools

Overall, you can see from the questions we have asked in this book, and those included in critical appraisal tools, that the questions we need to ask to assess rigour are fairly standard; there are more similarities than differences across study types. The more papers you read, the more you will recognise this. It is about thinking about the research (or review) question, then considering what approach was taken, what specific method was used, who the data was collected from, where it was collected and when and how (or, if a review, what papers were included), and thinking through the likely impact of the answers to these questions on the results and conclusions drawn by the authors.

Critical appraisal tools can help with this but, before you use an appraisal tool to assess a research paper, one important point to remember is that a tool won't help you understand the paper if you are not already familiar with the method. This is why we have explained the rationale for the steps taken in each research paper, identified key features for you to look out for and provided additional key reading at the end of each chapter. By focusing each chapter on a particular research or review paper, we hope this helps your understanding of key research concepts which you can then apply to other similar papers you read in the future.

References

Aveyard, H. (2019) *Doing a Literature Review in Health and Social Care* (4th edition). London: Open University Press.

Aveyard, H. and Bradbury-Jones, C. (2019) An analysis of current practice in undertaking literature reviews: A focussed mapping review and synthesis. *BMC Medical Research Methodology*, 19: 105.

Aveyard, H. and Sharp, P. (2017) *A Beginner's Guide to Evidence-based Practice* (3rd edition). London: Open University Press.

Aveyard, H., Payne, S. and Preston, N. J. (2021) *A Postgraduate's Guide to Doing a Literature Review in Health and Social Care* (2nd edition). London: Open University Press.

Barkway, P. (2001) Michael Crotty and nursing phenomenology: Criticism or critique. *Nursing Inquiry*, 8(3): 191–5.

Bazeley, P. (2009) Mixed methods data analysis. In S. Andrew and E. Halcomb (eds), *Mixed Methods Research for Nursing and the Health Sciences* (pp. 84–118). Chichester: Wiley-Blackwell.

Beauchamp, T. L. and Childress, J. F. (2001) *Principles of Biomedical Ethics* (5th edition). New York: Oxford University Press.

Benner, P. (1994a) Interpretive phenomenology. In P. Benner (ed.), *Interpretive Phenomenology: Embodiment, Caring and Ethics in Health and Illness* (pp. 99–127). Thousand Oaks, CA: Sage Publications.

Benner, P. (ed.) (1994b) *Interpretive Phenomenology: Embodiment, Caring, and Ethics in Health and Illness*. Thousand Oaks, CA: Sage Publications.

Blakey, E. P., Jackson, D., Walthall, H. and Aveyard, H. (2019) Memory in narratives and stories: Implications for nursing research. *Nurse Researcher*, 27(3): 27–32.

Braun, V. and Clarke, V. (2006) Using thematic analysis in psychology. *Qualitative Research in Psychology*, 3: 77–101.

Broome, M. E. (1993) Integrative literature reviews for the development of concepts. In B. L. Rodgers and K. A. Knafl (eds), *Concept Development in Nursing* (2nd edition, pp. 231–50). Philadelphia, PA: W. B. Saunders Co.

Charmaz, K. (2014) *Constructing Grounded Theory*. London: Sage Publications.

Christmals, C. D. and Gross, J. J. (2017) An integrative literature review framework for postgraduate nursing research reviews. *European Journal of Research in Medical Sciences*, 5: 7–15.

Cicco, M. A., Ragazzo, V. and Jacinto, T. (2016) Mortality in relation to the British Doctor's Study. *Breathe*, 12(3): 275–6.

Cochrane, A. L. (1972) *Effectiveness and Efficiency: Random Reflections on Health Services*. London: Nuffield Trust.

Colaizzi, P. (1978) Psychological research as a phenomenologist views it. In R. S. Valle and M. King (eds) *Existential Phenomenological Alternatives for Psychology*. New York: Open University Press.

Creswell, J. W. and Plano Clark, V. L. (2011) *Designing and Conducting Mixed Methods Research* (2nd edition). Thousand Oaks, CA: Sage Publications.

Crotty, M. (1996) *Phenomenology and Nursing Research*. Philadelphia, PA: W. B. Saunders Co.

Cutcliffe, J. R. and McKenna, H. P. (1999) Establishing the credibility of qualitative research findings: The plot thickens. *Journal of Advanced Nursing*, 30(2): 374–80.

Ellis, P. (2020) *Understanding Ethics for Nursing Students* (3rd edition). London: Learning Matters.

Elo, S. and Kyngäs, H. (2008) The qualitative content analysis process. *International Journal of Nursing Studies*, 62(1): 107–15.

General Medical Council (GMC) (2013) *Good Practice in Research*. London: GMC.

Giorgi, A. (ed.) (1985) *Phenomenology and Psychological Research*. Pittsburgh, PA: Duquesne University Press.

Glaser, B. G. and Strauss, A. (1967) *The Discovery of Grounded Theory*. Chicago: Aldine.

Guyatt, G. H., Oxman, A. D., Montori, V., Vist, G., Kunz, R., Brozek, J., ... & Schünemann, H. J. (2011) GRADE guidelines: 5. Rating the quality of evidence–publication bias. *Journal of Clinical Epidemiology*, 64(12): 1277–82.

Hagens, V., Dobrow, M. J. and Chafe, R. (2009) Interviewee transcript review: Assessing the impact on qualitative research. *BMC Medical Research Methodology*, 9(47): 1–8.

Hancock, S., Preston, N., Jones, H. and Gadoud, A. (2019) Telehealth in palliative care is being described but not evaluated: A systematic review. *BMC Palliative Care*, 18: article no. 114.

Higgins, J. P. T., Thomas, J., Chandler, J., Cumpston, M., Li, T., Page, M. J. and Welch, V. A. (eds) (2019) *Cochrane Handbook for Systematic Reviews of Interventions* (2nd edition). Chichester: John Wiley & Sons.

Jonsdottir, H., Amundadottir, O., Gudmundsson, G., Halldorsdottir, B., Hrafnkels-son, B., Ingadottir, T. S., Jonsdottir, R., Jonsson, J. S., Sigurjonsdottir, E. and Stefansdottir, I. (2015) Effectiveness of a partnership-based self-management programme for patients with mild and moderate chronic obstructive pulmonary disease: A pragmatic randomized controlled trial. *Journal of Advanced Nursing*, 71(11): 2634–49.

Krejcie, R. V. and Morgan, D. W. (1970) Determining sample size measurement for research activities. *Educational and Psychological Measurement*, 30(3).

Kvale, S. and Brinkmann, S. (2009) *Interviews: Learning the Craft of Qualitative Research Interviewing* (2nd edition). London: Sage.

Leonard, V. W. (1994) A Heideggerian phenomenological perspective on the concept of person. In P. Benner (ed.), *Interpretive Phenomenology: Embodiment, Caring and Ethics in Health and Illness* (pp. 43–62). Thousand Oaks, CA: Sage Publications.

Lincoln, Y. S. and Guba, E. G. (1985) *Naturalistic Inquiry*. Beverly Hills, CA: Sage Publications.

Malterud, K., Siersma, V. D. and Guassora, A. D. (2016) Sample size in qualitative interview studies: Guided by information power. *Qualitative Health Research*, 26(13): 1753–60.

Merleau-Ponty, M. (1945/2012) *The Phenomenology of Perception*. Abingdon: Routledge.

Moher, D., Liberati, A., Tetzlaff, J., Altman, D. G. and PRISMA Group (2009) Preferred reporting items for systematic reviews and meta-analyses: The PRISMA statement. *Journal of Clinical Epidemiology*, 62(10): 1006–12.

Moustakas, C. (1994) *Phenomenological Research Methods*. Thousand Oaks, CA: Sage Publications.

Nijjar, S. K., D'Amico, M. I., Wimalaweera, N. A., Cooper, N., Zamora, J. and Khan, K. S. (2017) Participation in clinical trials improves outcomes in women's health: A systematic review and meta-analysis. *BJOG*, 126(6): 863–71.

O'Cathain, A., Murphy, E. and Nicholl, J. (2008) The quality of mixed methods studies in health services research. *Journal of Health Services Research and Policy*, 13(2): 92–8.

O'Cathain, A., Murphy, E. and Nicholl, J. (2010) Three techniques for integrating data in mixed methods studies. *British Medical Journal*, 341: c4587.

Prochaska, J. O., Norcross, J. C. and DiClemente, C. C. (1994) *Changing for Good*. New York: William Morrow.

Ranse, T., Arbon, P., Cusack, L., Shabon, R. and Nicolls, D. (2020) Obtaining individual narratives and moving to an intersubjective lived experience description: A way of doing phenomenology. *Qualitative Research*, 20(6): 945–59.

Richards, D. A., Hanssen, T. A. and Borglin, G. (2018) The second triennial systematic literature review of European nursing research: Impact on patient outcomes and implications for evidence based practice. *Worldviews on Evidence Based Nursing*, 5(5): 333–43.

Richards, D. A., Hilli, A., Pentecost, C., Goodwin, V. A. and Frost, J. (2018) Fundamental nursing care: A systematic review of the evidence on the effect of nursing care interventions for nutrition, elimination, mobility and hygiene. *Journal of Clinical Nursing*, 27(11–12): 2179–88.

Sackett, D. L., Rosenberg, W. M. C., Gray, J. A. M., et al. (1996) Evidence-based medicine: What it is and what it isn't. *British Medical Journal*, 312: 71–2.

Sackett, D. L., Straus, S., Richardson, S., Rosenberg, W. and Haynes, R. B. (2000) *Evidence-based Medicine: How to Practice and Teach EBM*. London: Churchill Livingstone.

Sinclair, M., O'Toole, J., Malawaraarachchi, M. and Leder, K. (2012) Comparison of response rates and cost effectiveness for a community-based survey: Postal, internet and telephone modes with generic or personalised recruitment approaches. *BMC Medical Research Methodology*, 12: article no. 132.

Stolley, J. M., Buckwalter, K. C. and Garand, L. (2000) The evolution of nursing research. *Journal of Neuromusculoskeletal Systems*, 8(1): 10–15.

Tang, T. L. and Chiu, R. K. (2003) Income, money, ethics, pay satisfaction, commitment and unethical behaviour: Is love of money the root of all evil for Hong Kong employees? *Journal of Business Ethics*, 46(1): 13–30.

Tingen, M. S., Burnett, A. H., Murchison, R. B. and Zhu, H. (2009) The importance of nursing research. *Journal of Nursing Education*, 48(3): 167–70.

Twycross, A. and Shorten, A. (2014) Service evaluation, audit and research: What is the difference? *Evidence-Based Nursing*, 17: 65–6.

Urquhart, B., MacLehose, H. and Foxlee, R. (2017) A database to record the impact of fraud and misconduct in studies included in systematic reviews. https://abstracts.cochrane.org/2017-global-evidence-summit/database-record-impact-fraud-and-misconduct-studies-included-systematic

van Manen, M. (2017) But is it phenomenology? *Qualitative Health Research*, 27(6): 775–9.

West, R. and Brown, J. (2013) *Theory of Addiction* (2nd edition). Chichester: Wiley Blackwell.

Whittemore, R. and Knafl, K. (2005) The integrative review; updated methodology. *International Journal of Nursing Studies*, 52(5): 546–53.

Windfuhr, J. P. (2016) Indications for tonsillectomy stratified by the level of evidence. *GMS Current Topics in Otorhinolaryngol Head and Neck Surgery*, 15: 9.

Index

Page numbers in *italics* refer to figures; page numbers in **bold** refer to tables.